WHY SOME PEOPLE ALMOST ALWAYS STAY HEALTHY

INVESTIGATING ESSENTIAL OILS FOR BEGINNERS

Tonny M Ford, RN, BSN, PHN.

2015

WHY SOME PEOPLE ALMOST ALWAYS

Stay Healthy

INVESTIGATING ESSENTIAL OILS FOR BEGINNERS

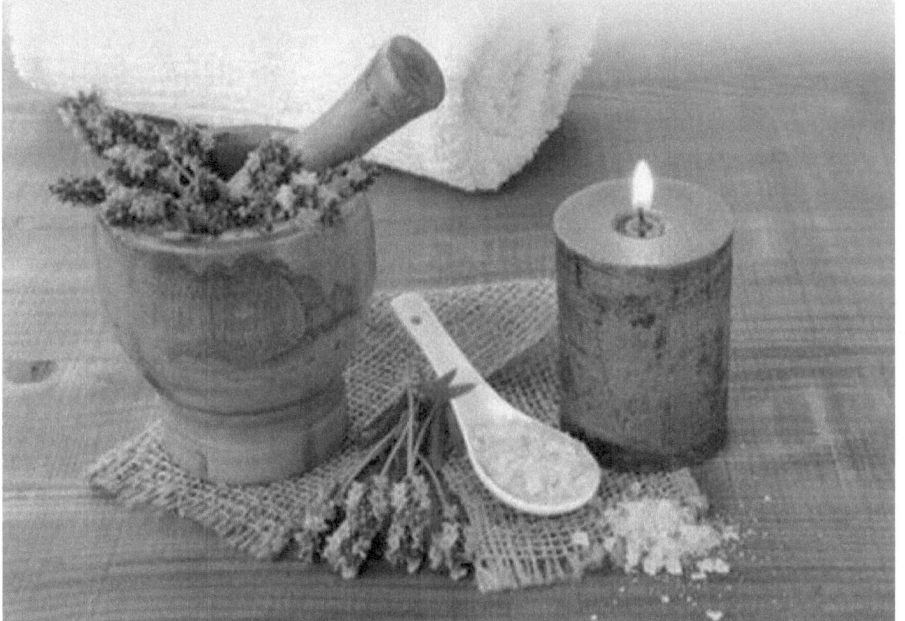

TONNY M FORD, RN, BSN, PHN

essentialoilRN.net

DISCLAIMER

This book is not intended as a substitute for the medical advice of physicians. The reader should regularly consult a physician in matters relating to his/her health and particularly with respect to any symptoms that may require diagnosis or medical attention.

The information provided in this book is designed to provide helpful information on the subjects discussed. This book is not meant to be used, nor should it be used, to diagnose or treat any medical condition. For diagnosis or treatment of any medical problem, consult your own physician. The publisher and author are not responsible for any specific health or medical needs that may require medical supervision and are not liable for any damages or negative consequences from any treatment, action, application or preparation, to any person reading or following the information in this book. References are provided for informational purposes only and do not constitute endorsement of

This document is geared towards providing exact and reliable information in regards to the topic and issue covered. The publication is sold with the idea that the publisher is not required to render accounting, officially permitted, or otherwise, qualified services. If advice is necessary, legal or professional, a practiced individual in the profession should be ordered.

- From a Declaration of Principles which was accepted and approved equally by a Committee of the American

presentation of the information is without contract or any type of guarantee assurance.

The trademarks that are used are without any consent, and the publication of the trademark is without permission or backing by the trademark owner. All trademarks and brands within this book are for clarifying purposes only and are the owned by the owners themselves, not affiliated with this document.

We highly recommend that you consult a doctor and other trained clinicians before using essentials oils or anything that can affect your health. Your doctor is the only one who knows the true story of your health and can give your better professional help.

TABLE OF CONTENTS

INTRODUCTION

My father took down some bottles from over the fireplace and mixed several liquids in a bowl. He then made a compress by folding a small piece of flannel, soaked it in the liquid, and placed it on the man's side. Within half an hour, the pains had gone, and his face was no longer screwed up out of all recognition as it had been. Gripping the table in my excitement, I couldn't take my eyes off him. It was a miracle!!

"Papa, did you do that?!"

"Mon cheri, he who causes the plants to grow is the one who did it."

Of Men and Plants

Maurice Messegue

I am always fascinated by the interesting question the kid asked his or her father. In my endeavors with essential oils, I can relate to this child. Assuming this kid is grown and now a renowned doctor, he would now say, "Most allopathic doctors think practitioners of alternative medicine are all quacks. They're not. Often they're sharp people who think differently about disease."

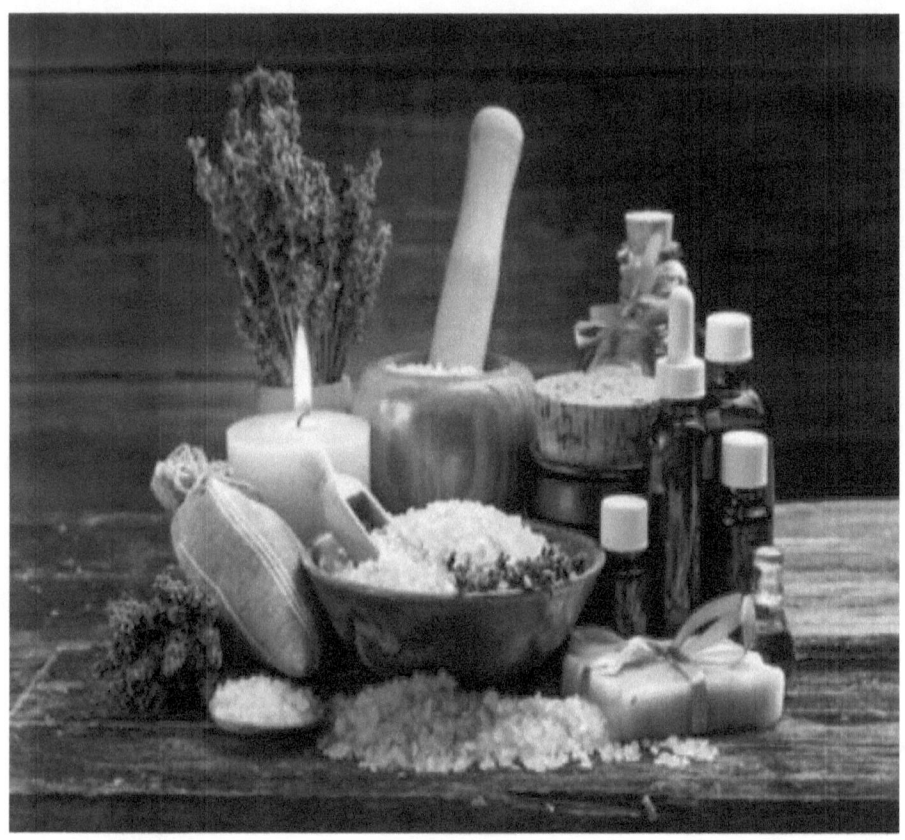

-Dr. Mehmet Oz

Essential oils are wonderful plant extracts that can benefit you and promote health and wellness, if used correctly. Just with any other alternative therapies, you cannot know if it works for you, unless you try. In this ebook, we have simple tips and strategies than anyone can use to empower themselves with sufficient knowledge to make an informed decision.

Are you interested in effective natural home remedies for a variety of health conditions? Would you like to begin using essential oils safely and effectively? Or do you just want more information on therapeutic essential oils?

If so, then this book is perfect for you.

Written to offer a comprehensive coverage of therapeutic essential oils, the book explains in amazing details what essential oils are, their history of usage, production, cycles of growth, application methods, dilutions, therapeutic properties, types of conditions treated, safety considerations, and purchasing of authentic and pure essential oils. While the book is not intended for diagnosing and prescribing essential oils for different ailments, it contains valuable educational and specific information on therapeutic uses of essential oils and will lead you into informed decision-making when you buy and use the oils.

So why is this book great?

(1)It gives comprehensive coverage of various topics in therapeutic usage of essential oils.

(2)It is a step-by-step guide to essential oils from definition to buying and using them.

(3)It has demystified ingestion (internal application) of essential oils.

(4)It covers the properties and uses of specific essential oils more broadly.

(5)It has prioritized the safety of users and offered a whole chapter on safety issues.

Once you have read this book, it is important to apply the information along with the guidance of a competent naturopathic professional. Moreover, as discussed in this book, internal consumption of essential oils must not be undertaken without the advice of a competent professional.

Finally, you have probably managed this far in your life without using essential oils and you may probably manage another week or more, as you read the material contained in this book and determine the right essential oils and correct dosages for you before you can begin using the oils. Therefore, I urge you to take your time to grasp as much information as possible so you can use essential oils sensibly, consistently, and safely.

I hope this book will help you to enjoy using essential oils!

CHAPTER 1: WHAT ARE ESSENTIAL OILS?

Essential oils is a collective term referring to liquids that are extracted from stems, seeds, leaves, roots, bark, and flowers of plants and distilled by means of steam or water to form highly-concentrated and volatile fluids with strong aroma. By definition, essential oils are concentrated hydrophobic liquids, containing volatile aromatic compounds from plants. They are called "Essential" because they contain the "true essence of plant fragrances" that are the characteristic fragrances of the plants from which they have been derived. Essential oils are also called Volatile Oils, Ethereal Oils, Aetherolea, or, simply, the "Oil of" the plants from which they have been extracted (such as Oil of Lavender and Oil of Clove).

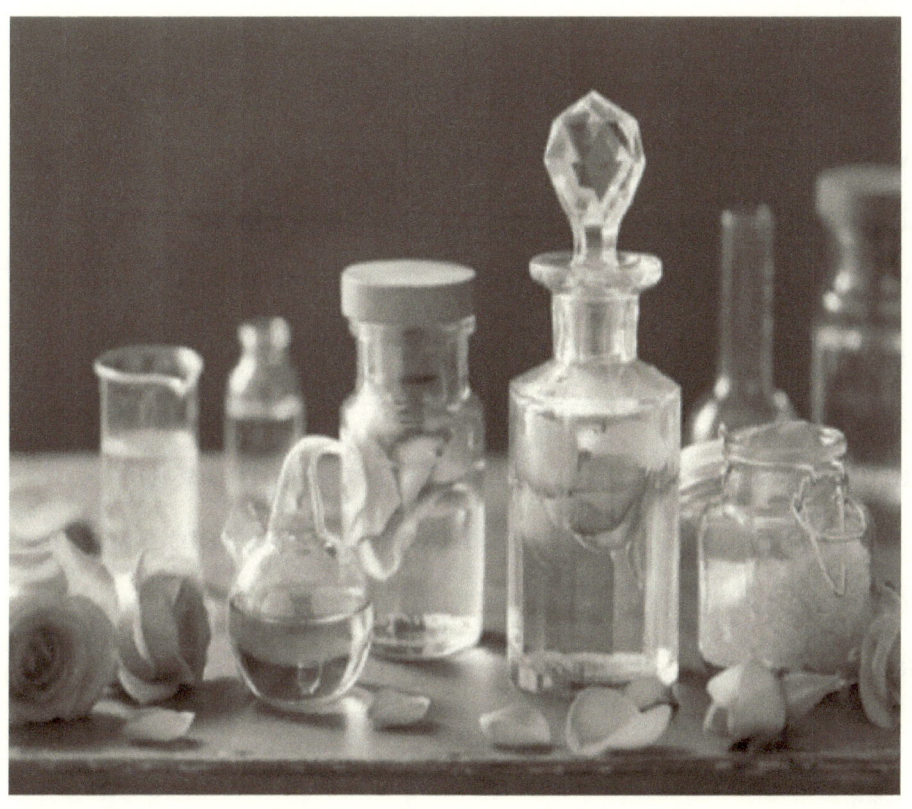

Extracted and distilled using a variety of methods
capable of capturing scented particles and leaving
behind other chemical constituents of plants, the oils
contain hundreds of organic compounds, such as
vitamins, hormones, and other natural elements, which
work on many levels. During extraction and
distillation, the most powerful healing compounds of a
plant are concentrated to form a liquid that is usually

75-100 times more concentrated than the oils in dried herbs.

Typically, essential oils are beneficial compounds, which play crucial roles in helping plants to survive in their natural habitats. The oils protect plants from insects, help them to adapt to their surroundings, and shield them from harsh environmental conditions. Composed of small molecules that can penetrate the human cells and change the chemical composition and physiology of the cells, essential oils have remarkable therapeutic value. Besides, many essential oils have some compounds that can cross the blood-brain barrier and influence brain function.

Like pure jewelry (or fine wine), essential oils are gems of nature. They are the quintessential life force borne by aromatic plants with every drop of the oils worth savoring, protecting, and enjoying. They are easily absorbed into the extracellular fluids of the cells beneath the surface of the skin to give a variety of effects, including nourishing, cleansing, balancing, and rejuvenating effects. They also diffuse perfectly into the air to deliver amazing olfactory benefits.

The majority of essential oils in the market have a clear color and consistency. However, there are some essential oils, such as lemongrass, orange, and patchouli, which can be amber or warm yellow. Nonetheless, the core characteristic of essential oils is that they have real and true essence regardless of the plants they are extracted from. And, since the oils are incredibly highly concentrated, small drops of the oils can give significant therapeutic value.

Moreover, essential oils differ from fatty oils (such as nut and vegetable oils), which contain larger molecules that cannot penetrate into human cells and therefore have no therapeutic value. Likewise, essential oils are not the same as perfumes or fragrance oils. While perfumes are usually artificially created and infused with fragrances and appealing smells in order to produce superficial effects, essential oils have natural scents and chemical compounds that offer therapeutic benefits.

HOW DO ESSENTIAL OILS WORK?

While medicinal use of essential oils is still considered as pseudoscience in the mainstream healthcare community, the oils retain considerable popularity among advocates of alternative medicine. Because of this, it has been difficult to obtain reliable references and studies on the pharmacological merits of essential oils. Nevertheless, the tide is beginning to change and more scientific studies on essential oils are being conducted around the globe. For instance, major clinical studies are currently underway in Australia, Japan, India, Canada, the United States, and Europe. Indeed, since 2000, there have been a growing number of publications on essential oils in traditional medical journals with over 1045 PubMed listed articles on essential oils in 2013 alone. The studies describe amazing healing properties of various oils, including effectiveness in treating pain, anxiety, infections, tumors, depression, nausea, postmenstrual syndrome, and more. Studies have also indicated that essential oils have the ability to prevent the transmission of a number of drug-resistant strains of pathogens, including Candida, streptococcus, and staphylococcus species.

So how do essential oils work? The oils contain minute molecules that are easily absorbed by the cells of the human body, resulting in therapeutic effects. Every essential oil, having a unique chemical composition of esters, alcohols, terpenes, ketones, aldehydes, oxides, and phenols, will therefore interact differently with bodily systems. Depending on the type of oil and its chemical composition, there will be stimulation of the immune system, elimination of toxins, enhanced cell growth, and death or inactivation of bacteria, viruses, fungi and parasites, among other activities. The actions of the chemical components of essential oils include:

a. Esters have anti-inflammatory, anti-viral, anti-fungal, anti-bacterial, and calming effects.

b. Aldehydes have sedative, anti-infectious, calming when inhaled, and topical irritation effects.

c. Ketones loosen mucous, stimulate cell regeneration, and have cleansing properties.

d. Phenols have antiseptic, anti-bacterial, fragrant, and anti-cancerous effects.

e. Alcohols, which stimulate the immune system, have anti-viral, antiseptic, and anti-bacterial effects.

f. Oxides have anesthetic, antiseptic, and expectorant effects.

g. Terpenes and Sesquiterpenes inhibit toxin accumulation and promote the discharge of toxins from the kidneys and liver. They cross blood-brain barrier; have antiseptic and anti-inflammatory properties; carry oxygen molecules into cells and throughout the body; and boost healing, memory, and immune system.

h. Farnesene, which is useful in re-balancing the digestive tract, has antiviral and antibacterial activities.

i. Limonene is found in citrus oils, which are antiviral and help with herpes simplex virus and other viruses.

j. Pinene, which is strongly antiseptic, is commonly found in Conifer oils, such as Fir, Spruce, Pine, and Juniper Berry.

For example, Lavender essential oils have 40 percent linalyl acetate, which is a powerful ester with anti-inflammatory, anti-bacterial, sedative, and anti-viral effects. Therefore, Lavender is the perfect oil for treating sleep disorders and for first aid. Similarly, because of their chemical components, Sandalwood oil and Frankincense oil are used to prevent cancer because they contribute to the death of cancer cells. Eucalyptus oil is used to treat influenza, colds, and respiratory infections, such as sinusitis and rhinitis, because it has anti-viral, anti-fungal, and anti-bacterial components. Tea Tree Oil (Melaleuca) is used to treat head lice. Essential oils, such as Lavender, Geranium, Grapefruit, Tea Tree, and Patchouli, have anti-bacterial properties and are, therefore, used for treating MRSA infections.

In fact, keeping the most common essential oils, such as Lemon, Frankincense, Peppermint, and Lavender in your natural medicine cabinet can help you to:

(i)   Relax your body.

(ii)   Soothe your muscles.

(iii)   Heal skin conditions.

(iv)   Fight flu and cold symptoms.

(v)   Alleviate pain.

(vi)   Improve your digestion.

(vii)   Balance hormones.

(viii) Reduce wrinkles and cellulite.

(ix)   Clean your home and keep bugs away.

Here are the most popular essential oils and how to use them:

a. Basil: Has analgesic, antispasmodic, and ophthalmic properties. It is used for treating indigestion, reducing stress, treating skin conditions, improving blood circulation problems, easing nausea, and treating respiratory problems.

b. Black Pepper: Treats a number of ailments, including bacterial infections, cramps, and joint pains.

c. Cypress: Enhances blood circulation, prevents varicose veins, boosts confidence, and promotes the healing of broken bones.

d. Clove: Has antioxidant, anti-parasitic, and anti-bacterial properties.

e. Frankincense: Reduces inflammation, boosts immunity, supports the brain, fights cancer, and heals aging spots.

f. Eucalyptus: Invigorates and purifies the body and improves respiratory conditions, such as allergies, sinusitis, and bronchitis.

g. Grapefruit: Reduces cellulite and supports metabolism. It is mixed with coconut and rubbed externally on areas with cellulite; or a few drops of the oil can be mixed with water and taken internally.

h. Geranium: It is commonly used to reduce the symptoms of PMS, refresh the skin, treat skin conditions (like acne), eliminate skin blemishes and light scars, and reduce inflammation.

i. Ginger: Supports joints, relieves nausea, improves digestion, and reduces inflammation.

j. Lemon: Cleanses the body and boosts lymph drainage. It can also be added to homemade cleaning products to boost their effectiveness.

k. Lavender: Improves mood, relaxes the body and mind, and heals cuts, burns, and wounds.

l. Myrrh: It is a natural antiseptic capable of preventing or reducing infections. It reduces body stretch marks, enhances hormone balance, and supports beautiful skin.

m. Peppermint: Boosts focus, supports digestion, reduces fever, boosts energy, and relieves headaches and muscle pain.

n. Pine: Has analgesic and antiseptic properties; treats skin conditions such as acne and eczema; eases joint pain; boosts metabolism; improves the symptoms of flu and cold; and kills germs.

o. Oregano: Has powerful anti-microbial properties and helps to kill fungi and treat colds.

p. Rosemary: Improves hair thickness and is usually added to homemade hair shampoos. It also enhances memory and brain function and is ideal for those who are reading, studying, or working routinely.

q. Rose: Has powerful anti-inflammatory effects and is used to reduce skin inflammation and create glowing skin. A few drops of the oil are usually added to facial moisturizers. It is recognized as the beautiful feminine oil and helps with hormonal balance. It eases the effects of menopause and PMS and improves the overall appearance of the skin.

r. Sesame: The oil contains fatty acids that help to reduce stress levels and lower blood pressure. It also slows the growth of cancer cells and has remarkable moisturizing qualities.

s. Sandalwood: The oil is a natural aphrodisiac, which boosts libido and improves energy levels.

Moreover, different essential oils can be blended together in order to boost their effectiveness. For example, the following conditions can effectively be treated with the highlighted essential oil combinations:

a. Occasional Throbbing Headaches: Apply a blend of Basil, Frankincense, and Soothing Blend to the back of your neck and temples.

b. Scrapes and Cuts: Apply 1 drop of Clove and 1 drop of Lavender directly to the wound and rub gently.

c. Sleeplessness: Rub a few drops of Lavender and Calming Blend to your feet just before going to bed.

d. To Boost Mental Focus: Diffuse Wild Orange or Citrus Bliss in your room or keep the oil at your desk.

e. Stomach Upset: Rub a few drops of Digestive Blend on your stomach.

f. Improving Immunity: Rub a few drops of Frankincense, Lemon and Melaleuca on your feet.

ARE ESSENTIAL OILS REALLY EFFECTIVE?

Generally, there are two opposite extremes to the usage of essential oils. One camp claims that essential oils are magic cures that can cure every condition under the sun; can fully replace conventional medicines; and care for mental and physical health problems. And, there is another camp that dismisses the whole idea of using essential oils as a filthy scam that is perpetuated by people who are either ill-informed or ill-intentioned towards duping the masses. Well, the truth lies squarely between these two extremes.

While essential oils have a long history of use and reliability in treating many health conditions and solving a litany of problems, they must never take the place of nutrient dense diets and conventional treatments. In fact, well-made essential oils should be used complimentarily with other therapeutic procedures in order to attain complete recovery and promote better health. Indeed, when the oils are combined with proper diets, they can quickly treat acute conditions, such as rashes, headache, respiratory problems, viral, and bacterial infections. They can even benefit people with autoimmune diseases and cancers.

Today, it is firmly recognized that most essential oils are effective and can be used in different settings as a form of non-invasive treatment for various medical conditions. The oils have curative effects when used in oil burners, massages, or diffused in the air through nebulizers. Similarly, diluted essential oils can be taken internally, inhaled, or applied to the body through baths. The oils may also be added to soaps, cosmetics, household cleaning products, other hygiene products, and in flavoring foods and drinks. In fact, many traditional hospitals, such as Vanderbilt University Hospital, are exploiting the therapeutic effects of essential oils and using the oils to treat depression, anxiety, infections in hospitalized patients, and other infections. Indeed, according to a 2009 study, pre-operative patients who were treated with the essential oil Lavandin felt less anxious about their impending surgeries than controls; while other oils, such as Lavender, Neroli, and Sandalwood were also shown to help patients to manage anxiety well.

The effectiveness of essential oils has also been confirmed in studies of their effects in midwifery. For example, according to a 2007 study published in the *Journal of Alternative and Complimentary Medicine*, women who used certain essential oils during labor reported that they experienced less pain, less anxiety, and less fear during childbirth, and were able to use minimal pain medications. Likewise, essential oils with anti-viral, anti-fungal, and anti-bacterial properties have been tested in medical settings and found effective. For example, it has been shown that when certain essential oils are massaged on the skin with burns, scrapes, or cuts, the skin conditions heal quickly. Other essential oils have been reported to aid in digestion, boost immunity, and help with insomnia. Moreover, there are numerous studies that have demonstrated that the use of Frankincense helps to shrink brain tumors and fight cancer.

MAXIMIZING EFFECTIVENESS OF ESSENTIAL OILS

Essential oils are typically very concentrated. Therefore, their safe and effective use requires handling them with great care and respect; taking time to learn about the properties and effects of the oils before using them; and prioritizing the application of drops rather ounces. In order to maximize the benefits of essential oils, you should:

a. Always read label precautions, warnings, and instructions carefully and follow them to the letter. Every bottle of essential oil comes labeled with directions on how to use the oil. Make sure to check the product label for appropriate usage directions before you apply the oil.

b. Keep your essential oils in tightly closed containers and out of the reach of children.

c. Never ingest any essential oil unless the usage directions indicate that the oil can be used internally.

d. Never use essential oils on your skin without dilution. It is prudent to dilute oils with proper recommended vegetable oils, such as Grapeseed oil or sweet almond oil.

e. Conduct skin tests for every essential oil before applying on your skin. To achieve this, simply dilute a small quantity of the oil and apply the diluted portion to the skin of your inner arm. If irritation or redness occurs, do not use that oil on your skin.

f. Keep essential oils away from your mucous membranes and eyes.

g. When you experience itching, irritation, burning, or redness after applying any essential oil to your skin, stop using that oil immediately.

h. Angelica and all citrus oils cause skin sensitivity to ultraviolet light. Therefore, you must avoid going out into the sun after applying such oils to your skin.

i. Individuals with high blood pressure MUST avoid using thyme, sage, rosemary, and hyssop oils.

j. Individuals with leprosy MUST avoid using sage, rosemary, hyssop, and sweet funnel oil.

Skin irritation or discomfort is one of the most common problems associated with using essential oils. Whenever you experience irritation or discomfort, you must stop using the essential oil and apply carrier oil to the irritated area immediately. You must never use water to flush off the oil from your skin because this can increase the discomfort. If you experience a skin rash, this may indicate detoxification, and it is advised that you drink plenty of water to encourage the removal of the toxins from your body.

Additionally, since toxins in petrochemical-based products, such as soaps, detergents, perfumes, and skin care products usually trigger detoxification reactions, you should discontinue the use of such products as soon as skin reaction occurs. Before using the same essential oil that caused a reaction previously, conduct a patch test and then dilute the oil with carrier oil as necessary. And, if any essential oil gets into your eye, flush it off with carrier oil in order to alleviate the discomfort. But if the discomfort fails to subside within five minutes, then seek medical attention.

FREQUENCY AND QUANTITY OF USING ESSENTIAL OILS

How often should you apply essential oils and how much should you use? The proper frequency and quantity of essential oil you should use is indicated on the label. Make sure to follow the label directions carefully and to avoid the temptation to use more than the quantity indicated. Remember that essential oils are powerful and potent and must be started on slowly and increased gradually depending on the results. Most often, 1-2 drops of the essential oil is enough and using more than this is often a waste of the product.

And, depending on the type of essential oil, you should apply it 3-4 times per day. Avoid excessive application of the oils, as this will increase the risks of adverse reactions. As well, essential oils must never come into direct contact with sensitive areas, such as the genitals, ears, mucous membranes, and eyes. But, if there is an overwhelming need to use essential oils in a sensitive area, make sure to dilute the oils at a ratio of 1 drop of the oil to 5-10 drops of the carrier oil.

CARRIER OILS AND HOT OILS

Carrier oil is typically a vegetable oil, such as sweet almond oil, coconut oil, avocado oil, or grapeseed oil, which can be used to dilute an essential oil. By adding carrier oils to essential oils, the concentration of the essential oils is reduced to allow for their safe and comfortable application. Most importantly, however, the dilution by carrier oil does not diminish the effects or therapeutic value of the diluted essential oil and only serves to prevent wastage that may result from excessive application. Nevertheless, vegetable shortening, margarine, butter, and petroleum derivatives (such as petroleum jelly) must never be used as carrier oils; while olive oil may be avoided by those who are put off by its thick viscosity and strong aroma.

Hot oils are types of essential oils that can cause hot or burning sensations when applied to the skin. Therefore, when using hot oil for the first time, it is recommended that you do a patch test to determine how it affects your skin. To conduct a patch test, you only need to apply 1-2 drops of the hot essential oil to a patch of your skin (such as forearm) and observe the effects of the oil on the skin for 1-2 hours to see if there are any noticeable reactions. Usually, the reactions occur within 5 to 10 minutes, but it is prudent to wait for at least an hour to be certain about the effects of the essential oil. If you experience a burning (hot) sensation or develop a rash, then you should add carrier oil to the area as soon as the burning is experienced and as often as necessary. Examples of hot essential oils are clove, peppermint, thyme, thieves, lemongrass, cinnamon, Exodus II, and oregano.

PREGNANCY, CHILDREN AND CHRONIC MEDICAL CONDITIONS

Pregnant or nursing women must never use essential oils without first seeking the advice and recommendation of competent and trained health care practitioners who are experienced in essential oil usage. Besides, it is generally recommended that pregnant or nursing mothers must avoid excessive use of Hyssop (Hyssopus officinalis), Tansy (Tanacetum vulgare), Sage (Salvia officinalis), Wintergreen (Gaultheria procumbens), Fennel (Foeniculum vulgare), Clary Sage (Salvia sclarea), and all supplements and blends containing these oils. Moreover, the following oils should be avoided during pregnancy or nursing: clove bud, bitter almond, marjoram, clary sage, basil, sweet fennel, peppermint, myrrh, wintergreen, sage, rosemary, rose, juniper berry, hyssop, and thyme.

Many essential oils can safely be used with children. In fact, there are essential oil products that have been appropriately pre-diluted with carrier oils and are intended for applying directly on children. Nevertheless, since children usually respond well to essential oils, it is recommended that all the oils are sufficiently diluted prior to application. For example, 1-

2 drops of essential oil blends, like Gentle Baby, Peace & Calming, RutaVala, or SleepyIze, can be diluted with carrier oil and applied directly to the bottom of a child's feet.

For individuals with chronic medical conditions and those on prescription drugs, it is wise to consult health care experts with experience on usage of essential oils for recommendations and advice. Make sure to ask the prescribing physician and a pharmacist about the potential interactions between the medications you are taking and the essential oils prescribed. Furthermore, you should exercise caution, as you start using a new essential oil by conducting a patch test, diluting the oil adequately, and applying few drops of the oil.

CHAPTER 2: BRIEF HISTORY OF THE USE OF ESSENTIAL OILS

Earliest Uses of Essential Oils

The therapeutic effects of essential oils (EOs) have been known to many different cultures for over 5,000 years. Relying on the incredibly powerful sense of smell, the earliest human beings quickly identified various oils that could be used for different purposes. And, by experimenting with essential oils, they learned that different oils were great, natural, and potent treatments for a variety of health conditions. And, while it is difficult to point out where the practice of using healing plant oils first originated, many civilizations, including the Egyptians, Jews, Chinese, Greeks, Indians, and Romans, have historical records pointing to several centuries of using the oils as perfumes, cosmetics, and medicinal agents. In some cultures, essential oils were used in spiritual rituals.

The earliest evidence of usage of essential oils for therapeutic purposes was found in the Lascaux area of Dordogne in France. At Lascaux, cave paintings of medicinal plants used in treating various conditions were found and carbon dated back to 18,000 B.C.E. And, as early as 4500 B.C.E, Egyptians were using essential oils as part of different herbal preparations, perfumed oils, balsams, spices, resins, scented barks, and aromatic vinegars. For instance, Egyptians had a popular herbal preparation called "Kyphi," which contained 16 potent essential ingredients and was used as a perfume, incense, or medicine. Smoke and ashes from onion, cedar, aniseed, grapes, watermelon, and garlic were used for healing purposes; pastes and oils from plants were made into powders, pills, suppositories, ointments, and medicinal cakes; and aromatic gums, such as myrrh and cedar, were used for embalming. The most common essential oils used by Egyptians were myrrh, Frankincense, Spikenard, Elemi, Oregano, Rosemary, Nutmeg, Hyssop, Clove, Almond, Juniper, Henna, Galbanum, Cypress, Coriander, Cedarwood, Acacia, Cassia, Peppermint, Cinnamon, and Citronella.

Records of the use of essential oils in China date back to 2697 B.C.E. when the legendary Yellow Emperor, Huang Ti, ruled China. In his famous book of medicine, *The Yellow Emperor's Book of Internal Medicine*, Huang Ti describes several aromatic compounds and how they can be used to treat various conditions. The essential oils were classified into six groups, according to their mood-inducing properties, namely, luxurious, tranquil, noble, reclusive, refined, and beautiful. Following the expert writings of Emperor Huang Ti, the Chinese used essential oils to scent their bodies, clothes, hair, temples, and homes, while also producing sweet-smelling stationery, such as papers and inks. The Chinese book, *Materia Medica*, was the first comprehensive reference book describing the uses, healing properties, and proper preparation of more than 250 plant substances.

While no one knows exactly when Indian Traditional Medicine, Ayurveda, emerged, it is believed to have been practiced for more than 4000 years. Ayurveda is one of the oldest therapies with elaborate descriptions on disease pathways and the various techniques/methods and treatments for health disorders. More importantly, Ayurvedic literature dating from 2000 B.C.E contain records of Vedic Brahmans (sages/priests/physicians) administering the oils of myrrh, cinnamon, spikenard, coriander, and sandalwood to different patients. Since aromatic oils and plants were believed to be a godly part of nature and formed a critical part of the philosophical and spiritual outlook of Ayurvedic medicine, great effort was placed in describing how to use the oils carefully. In fact, 700 different aromatics and herbs have been described in the Vedas, the most sacred book of Hindus, including their uses is perfumes, religious aromatics, and healing agents. During the outbreak of Bubonic Plague, Ayurvedic principles were used successfully to replace ineffective antibiotics.

The flourishing trade between Egypt and Babylon in the 1800 B.C.E resulted in widespread use of essential oils for cosmetic and medicinal purposes. For instance, EOs, such as cedarwood, cypress, cinnamon, and myrrh, were traded on and used as antiseptics, air purification, body and hair treatments, pleasure aromas, incense, and ceremonial anointing. By 500 B.C.E, the Greeks had adopted the use of essential oils for medicinal purposes, with myrrh, cassia, cinnamon, frankincense, mint, thyme, marjoram, saffron, peppermint, and cumin being used for different purposes. The establishment of a medical school on the Greek Island of Cos was a landmark step in the expansion of the medicinal use of essential oils. For example, Hippocrates, the famous healer and "father of medicine," graduated from the school and advanced the use of perfumed baths and essential oil massages for keeping the body healthy and germ-free. The Greek physician, Megallus, developed a perfume brand made of a blend of essential oils and used it to treat wounds and reduce inflammation. Another Greek physician, Galen, used his knowledge of plant medicine and essential oils to heal post-surgical wounds and prevent wound infections. To avail the knowledge of plant medicine to Greeks and Romans, Dioscordes produced a catalogue of all the known herbs and their medicinal value in his comprehensive book, *De Materia Medica*. The book became a useful reference for Greeks and Romans, who extracted oils from plants and created different recipes with healing properties.

The Romans stretched the use of essential oils and aromatics to new heights. In self-indulgent Rome, communal bathing facilities were created not only for recreational purposes but also for healing and cosmetic reasons. Essential oil blends containing Cinnamon, Saffron, Myrrh, Calamus, Melissa, Spikenard, Orange, and Rose were used for body massages, scenting bed clothes, hair toning, and cosmetics. By 3AD, there were more than 1000 fragrant spas in the city of Rome, and aromatics were used for spiritual, cultural, and medicinal purposes. In fact, the popularity of aromatics by the time of the birth of Jesus Christ is alluded to in the Bible with the wise men being said to have carried the precious oils of myrrh and frankincense to the baby Jesus. Indeed, it was believed during those times that the incense of myrrh and frankincense kept away obsessions, anxieties, fears, and high-strung emotions. Later on, there is reference of Jesus' feet being anointed by Mary, using Spikenard, an expensive and cherished essential oil with therapeutic capacity. Of course, Spikenard enables a deep state of trancelike meditation and has regenerative properties that make it great for treating dry, tired, scaly-skinned calloused feet.

From Rome, the use of essential oils spread throughout the Roman Empire. During their conquests of the East and the North, the Romans spread their knowledge of the healing properties of essential oils to the Ancient Celts, Brits, and Nordics. But after the fall of the Roman Empire in the West, a great lull in the development of aromatherapy occurred. While trade in resins and spices remained robust between the East and the West, the amazing wealth of the healing power of essential oils was put aside. In fact, only the less lavish Gnostic Christians upheld the use of essential oils as a way of boosting their spirituality and helping their souls to go beyond the limitations of the material world and gain heavenly status. And, during the Dark Ages, the monks became the custodians of the knowledge of essential oils. In their monasteries, the monks created formal and raised herbal beds and prepared potent recipes for healing different health conditions. For example, Saint Hildegard, the Abbess of Bingen, was a renowned herbalist of the 12th century who produced 4 great works on the *Causes and Curses of Illness* and highlighted the efficacy of herbs in curing illnesses. Her favorite essential oil was Lavender.

Meanwhile, essential oils were a critical part of Arab cultures. For instance, during the 6th-7th centuries, fragrances of Rose and Henna were favorites in the Arab world. Rose water was used for scenting clothes, cleansing mosques, sweetening foods, and welcoming guests. The most notable advancement was made by Ali al-Husain Ibn (known in the West as Avicenna the Arab), who lived from 980-1037 A.D. Becoming a physician at the age of 12, Ali-Ibn wrote great books on the properties of over 800 plants and their effects on the human body. Ali-Ibn also created the first distillation technique for essential oils, which consisted of coiled pipes that allowed plant vapors and steam to cool down and delivered highly concentrated essential oils.

By the 13th century, Al-Samarqandi wrote elaborate essential oil recipes for powders, unguents, and baths, suggesting the use of dill, fennel, hyssop, mint, chamomile, thyme, and marjoram for treating sinus infections and ear problems. Around the same time, in 12the century India, Somershvara produced reliable writings on bathing rituals with essential oils and suggested the use of basil, cardamom, clove, coriander, jasmine, pine, saffron, agarwood, champac, costus, and pandanus in baths. Essential oils, such as musk, saffron, spikenard, amber, patchouli, and sandalwood, were to be applied on different body parts during tantric ceremonies.

The Renaissance and Beyond

At the dawn of the Renaissance, in the 1300s, trade in spices got a huge boost. The Crusades had provided the necessary contact with Arabic world and resulted in the rediscovery and usage of exotic herbs and essential oils in the West. Italy soon monopolized Eastern trade. The new wave of demand for spices quickly made Rose oil a hugely prized commodity and enabled Arabs to make huge profits of up to 300%. Shortly, Marco Polo journeyed to China in order to establish direct trade in spices and bypass the Moslem middleman; while Christopher Columbus set off to find other reliable sources of spices for Spain. By 1498, Vasco da Gama found his way around Africa to India, establishing direct trade in spices for Portugal. In fact, with direct access to such delights as pepper, ginger, cloves, and benzoin, Portugal shortly became the queen of spice trade, compelling Italy to persuade the Moslems into war with the Portuguese.

During the Renaissance, herbalists and alchemists categorized different essential oils, herbs, and plants according to their effects on the body. There was a predominant belief that the location, structure, shape, or appearance of a plant reflected its healing properties. For example, the leaves of Lungwort were used to treat lung complications because they looked like lungs. Similarly, Self Heal is shaped like the throat and was used to relieve tonsillitis, and leaves of the Kidneywort resemble the kidneys and were used for kidney problems. The colors of the plants also reflected their efficacy. For example, red plants, such as Coffee and Cinnamon, were believed to have stimulating effects; while blue plants, such as Roman Chamomile, were thought to have sedative qualities. Equally, yellow plants, such as Calendula, were used for relieving depression.

Furthermore, oils extracted from plant roots were thought to have grounding effects; those from hollow stems were thought to have clearing and opening effects; and those from solid stems were thought to give balance and stability. Oils from leaves were thought to cause ability to flow and flexibility; those from flowers were thought to boost spiritual growth and headiness; and those from whole plants were used as general tonics for the entire body. And, even though this kind of classification and usage of essential oils was often flawed, it rolled on the wheel of using the oils during the Renaissance and beyond.

In the 14th Century, the ravages of plague resulted in increased use of essential oils. Different essential oils were burned inside and outside of death houses to purify the air, and almost all aromatic herbs were used to combat Black Death. For example, a story is told of four thieves who used a blend of rosemary, cloves, lavender, and other essential oils in their face masks in order to enter and steal from the homes of those who were plagued. They knew that the essential oils had germ-killing properties and would kill the germs and protect them from infections during their exploits. In the 17th Century, Nicholas Culpeper developed his easy-to-understand tomes on herbal pharmacology to enable laypersons to use herbal remedies effectively. Nevertheless, by the late 17th Century, charlatanism sprung up, and Culpeper's knowledge of essential oils, recipes, and herbal formulas was misused and bastardized, resulting in diminished efficacy.

In 1910, René-Maurice Gattefosse, an accomplished French chemist, experimented with using Lavender oil to treat a burn on his hand. When the essential oil successfully healed the burn on his hand, he decided to conduct a comprehensive research on how to exploit the healing properties of Lavender oil to treat different conditions, such as burns, wounds, and skin infections. Indeed, by 1928, it was Gattefosse who pioneered the modern science of Aromatherapy and advanced the use of essential oils to treat many conditions. Initially, Gattefosse opted to prepare potent essential oil products for helping injured soldiers during the First World War (World War I), but the use of the oils was quickly picked up by different practitioners of alternative medicine (such as beauticians and massage therapists) and became popular throughout Europe.

While Gattefosse worked with essential oils and exploited the anti-microbial properties of the oils for different purposes, he influenced the practices of many physicians, the most notable one being Jean Valnet. Valnet was a Parisian medical doctor and army surgeon, and he quickly began to use essential oils for treating war wounds. During the Indochina War of 1948-1959, Valnet achieved great success in wound treatment and soon published a comprehensive text on aromatherapy in 1964, known as *Aromatherapie*, which earned him global recognition. During that time, Margaret Maury was working with Valnet, but she did not feel comfortable with the internal use of essential oils. As a biochemist, Margaret started experimenting with external application of essential oils and borrowed the massage techniques that had been taught by Micheline Arcier. Her aromatherapy massages achieved great success and laid the groundwork for most of the techniques used today.

In the 1980s, essential oils became core ingredients in lotions, candles, and fragrances. Similarly, a huge body of trained professionals, such as physical therapists, nutritionists, aromatherapists, and massage therapists, started recommending and using essential oils in their practices. For example, the French MD, Daniel Pénoël, worked with the French biochemist, Pierre Franchomme, to investigate and catalogue the medical properties of more than 270 essential oils and recommended their uses in the clinical environment. In 1990, the book *L'aromatherapie Exactement* was published in French and quickly became the primary reference for many secondary authors writing on the therapeutic uses of essential oils. Today, in Germany, England, and France, it is quite common for doctors to ask patients to choose between natural essential oils and prescription medicines, and both are distributed by pharmacies across Europe.

Chapter 3: APPLICATION METHODS FOR ESSENTIAL OILS

Essential oils have the capacity to alter our mental, physical, and emotional well-being by strengthening and triggering different natural processes in our bodies. The oils contain tiny molecules that can easily be absorbed by our body cells to deliver healing to various systems controlling our psychological, anatomical, and physiological states. Depending on the desired therapeutic effects, essential oils can be administered by a single or a combination of delivery methods. The method of delivery of any essential oil is usually chosen based on the aims of using the oil, the properties of the oil, and the safety concerns associated with the oil.

For easy recognition of how to use different essential oils, the degree of safety, and need for dilution, the following color symbols are used:

a. **GREEN**: Indicates that the essential oil is generally safe and can be used as directed without dilution.

b. **ORANGE**: Indicates that the essential oil requires moderate dilution and precautions.

c. **RED**: Indicates that the essential oil requires heavier dilution and precautions and that there is need to consult a naturopathic physician for advice on how to use it on the elderly, ill, children, and pregnant or nursing mothers.

Some essential oils, like peppermint and lemon, have many application methods while others, like wintergreen and its blends, have only one method of application. Therefore, it is critical to research every essential oil extensively in order to know the right method(s) of administration. Besides, it is worth remembering that the usage recommendations for essential oils are based only on high quality oils, which do not contain fillers and contaminants. Hence, it is important to buy top quality essential oils and use them according to the directions of the manufacturing company. For example, if the company does not recommend using the oil internally, do not try using the oil in that way.

When buying essential oils, you must remember there are no industry standards and regulations for the terms "pure" and "natural." In fact, many essential oil brands in drug stores may NOT be therapeutic grade and may even be low quality oils, containing adulterants and contaminants. Therefore, make sure to choose the oil you are buying carefully. The best essential oil brand should:

a. Be produced from proper plant varieties.

b. Have been grown without herbicides, pesticides, etc.

c. Have been grown indigenously.

d. Have been harvested with proper timing in order to ensure peak properties.

e. Have been extracted using proper pressure and temperature that preserved the oil molecules.

f. Have every batch taken through third-party testing.

There are eight fundamental guidelines on using essential oils:

a. **Personal Judgment:** Your judgment, self-belief, and trusting the abilities of your medical practitioner is the first step in learning and using essential oils safely and effectively. You understand your body better than anyone else, and, with little trial and error, you can quickly identify essential oils that suit your needs.

b. **Safe Does Not Mean Foolproof:** Every substance can be harmful to the body if used incorrectly. Even pure water can cause adverse effects when abused. Therefore, you must remember that essential oils are only safe when used appropriately, but they can cause adverse effects when used incorrectly. Before using the oils, make sure to know your sensitivities, health needs, and the properties and precautions of the EO that you are about to use. Ease yourself to the chemical components of the oil by diluting it properly, patch testing, and by starting with smaller amounts. Remember that most essential oil usage recommendations are for healthy adults, and anyone else (the elderly, sick, immuno-compromised, children, and pregnant women) must seek medical advice before using the oils.

c. **Follow Precautions Strictly and Wisely:** The label directions and precautions are usually provided to guide you into using essential oils appropriately and safely. While learning to use the oils correctly will take time and common sense, following precautions will minimize the risks involved. Make sure to start using the oils conservatively; apply less first and never overdo any application.

d. **Use Best Quality Essential Oils:** Some essential oils sold in drug stores are mixed with synthetic materials and other ingredients, which may cause adverse reactions. Therefore, make sure to choose a quality brand with a seed-to-seal guarantee and from a transparent manufacturer, who has clearly outlined the process of growing and producing the oil.

e. **Dilute Oils with carrier oils and not water:** Oils do not mix with water and must be diluted with the right vegetable oils. Essential oils MUST be diluted when they feel hot (warm) on the skin or when they have to be used over larger areas of the body (like back and legs). Dilution also prevents the oils from evaporating too quickly. Typically, every bottle of essential oil comes with a label, indicating the recommended dilution ratio. For instance, PanAway is diluted at a ratio of 1:4 (1 drop of PanAway with 4 drops of carrier oil). Dilution ratios may also be indicated as 50-50 (1 part of essential oil with 1 part of carrier oil) or 20-80 (1 part of essential oil with 4 parts of carrier oil), among others.

f. **Photosensitive Oils:** Some oils are photosensitive and must never be used on the skin that is frequently exposed directly to sunlight. Examples of such oils are Citrus Oils and Joy.

g. **You Are Unique:** Each person reacts differently to different essential oils. Therefore, make sure to conduct a patch test and to use a single essential oil at a time.

h. **Protect Your Ears and Eyes:** Ensure the essential oils do not get into them (ears and eyes).

Generally, there are 4 common ways of applying essential oils: topically, aromatically, ingestion, and externally (around the home).

TOPICAL APPLICATION OF ESSENTIAL OILS

The active ingredients in essential oils have smaller chemical weights of less than 1000 m (where m= weight of molecule). According to scientific theory and practice, any substances with molecular weights of 1000 m and below are easily absorbed by the skin. And, since the human skin is somewhat permeable, the essential oils usually penetrate the skin quickly and pass into the bloodstream before distributing to different areas of the body to deliver internal, therapeutic benefits.

Nevertheless, skin penetration is not as straightforward as it seems. Usually, the essential oils must enter and penetrate the stratum corneum (the thin outer skin layer), which is equipped for protecting the body against invasion by organisms. This presents a big challenge that may lead to 4 types of results after the oil is applied. Firstly, the essential oil may remain in the skin and become metabolized by cutaneous enzymes into carvacrol, methyl-carvacrol, safrole, and other substances. Secondly, the essence of the oil may remain in the skin and bind to the stratum corneum (or subcutaneous fat), forming a reservoir that releases the essence slowly into the capillaries. Thirdly, components of the essential oil might bind with proteins found in the skin, resulting in allergic contact dermatitis. Finally, the best-case scenario involves all or part of the essential oil being absorbed into the cutaneous micro-circulation.

The success of topical application of essential oils depends on optimal absorption of the oil applied in the cutaneous micro-circulation. Fortunately, the hair follicles, apocrine glands, and eccrine glands, which constitute 1% of the skin surface, usually provide easier access routes for the oils than the keratin and cellular components of the stratum corneum. In fact, some areas of the human skin (such as the palms, wrists, forehead, genitals, back of the neck, temples, head, under arms, mucous membranes, and soles of the feet) are more permeable than other areas of the skin and should be prioritized during topical essential oil application.

Skin permeability to essential oils can be increased by:

a. Altering the stratum corneum through abrasions, thinning of the layer, and cuts.

b. Hydrating the skin through bathing, sweating, or exposure to extra-humid environments (such as steam cabinet or steam room). For example, applying the oil on the skin after shower or after a hot bath will increase oil absorption because of increased blood flow to the dermis.

c. Using easily absorbed carrier oil (like fractionated coconut oil) instead of thicker slowly-absorbed carrier oil (like olive oil). Usually, oils with poly-saturated fats are more easily absorbed; while certain fatty acids contained in cold-pressed vegetable oils enhance skin permeability.

d. Covering the skin with a massage linen, wrap, clothing, or mask to inhibit evaporation and increase skin temperature. When covered, the skin will experience more hydration and more blood supply, resulting in increased permeability.

e. Using soap and other surfactants, such as aromatherapy shampoos, and shower gels, to increase the permeability of the skin.

f. Applying heat/warmth to the area of essential oil application to improve blood circulation and enhance the absorption of essential oil.

g. Massaging the target site for essential oil application before administering the oil to increase blood circulation on the area and cause increased absorption of the oils leading to quicker distribution and rapid action.

Even though most essential oils can be administered topically, usage varies from oil to oil. And, while some essential oils come with dilution and frequency precautions, it is important to remember that even those that do not come with such precautions can still affect some skin types adversely. This results in rashes or itchiness when not used with mindfulness. Essentially, therefore, you must know your skin type before using essential oils topically. And, if you have a sensitive skin, then you must always dilute the oils before usage, no matter the oil. Similarly, if your skin tends to be sensitive, then you must conduct a skin patch test on your inner arm before using the oils. Moreover, you should start with a single diluted drop and then top up with undiluted drops, if you are using essential oil that is generally safe for undiluted use by most people. Remember, also, to use one type of oil at a time for recognition of the oils that cause negative reactions on your skin.

CATEGORIES OF ESSENTIAL OILS FOR TOPICAL APPLICATION

There are three categories of oils for topical application, namely, neat, sensitive, and dilute.

a. **NEAT**: This category of oils can be applied to the skin undiluted. Nevertheless, it is still wiser to conduct a patch test on your skin every time you are using NEAT oil for the first time. And, because dilution will not hurt the therapeutic effects of the oil, it is a good idea to dilute the oil even if it is NEAT. Examples of NEAT oils are Frankincense, Lavender, Joy, Valor, Stress Away, and Purification.

b. **SENSITIVE**: This category of oils can be applied directly to the skin undiluted but MUST be diluted before use by persons with sensitive skin (the elderly and children). When diluting SENSITIVE oils, use the ratio 1:3 (1 drop of the oil to 3 drops of carrier oil).

c. **DILUTE**: This category of oils is very potent and MUST be diluted in the ratio 1:3 or more, depending on the skin sensitivity and age of the user. Using these oils undiluted can cause serious skin irritation and may be dangerous for nursing and pregnant women. In fact, the oils should not be used on children and must only be used by pregnant (or nursing women), the elderly, and the ill after consulting naturopathic doctors and after very high dilution. Examples include Thieves, Peppermint, PanAway, Lemon, and Peace & Calming.

While some essential oils are NEAT and can be applied to the skin directly without diluting with carrier oils, it is generally recommended that all essential oils be diluted with appropriate vegetable oil (such as coconut oil, almond oil or olive oil) before applying to the skin. Besides, it is prudent to conduct a skin patch test when using any essential oil for the first time. Moreover, extra caution should be exercised when applying essential oils to babies and small children. And it is also wise to dilute the oils thoroughly with carrier oils before applying on babies and children. Furthermore, menthol-containing oils (such as camphor, peppermint, and eucalyptus) must be used cautiously with children and must never be applied around the face.

Common examples of topically applied oils include German Chamomile (Matricaria recutita), which is used to treat eczema; Ginger (Zinziber officinalis), which is applied to improve flexibility and reduce arthritis pain; and black pepper (Piper nigrum).

WHERE TO APPLY ESSENTIAL OILS TOPICALLY

1. **Vita Flex Points:** Vita Flex is a short form for "Vitality through the Reflexes." The most common Vita Flex points for topical application are found at the bottoms of the feet and in both the hands. For example, if you want to use peppermint to improve your digestion, you can mix 1 drop of the oil with 1 drop of carrier oil and then apply the mixture to the Vita Flex point for digestion/stomach that is found in the left foot.

2. **Direct application to the affected area:** Essential oils are effective when applied directly to the affected areas. For example, the peppermint mixture in (1) above can be applied directly to the stomach surface instead of the feet.

3. **Forehead and Temples:** If you want to relax your mind, then you should apply the right essential oils (such as Lemon, Peppermint, or Lavender) to your forehead and temples.

4. **Back of the Neck and Bridge of the Nose:** If you want relief from seasonal sniffles, then you can apply the right essential oil (such as Lemon,

Peppermint, or Lavender) to the back of your neck and to the bridge of your nose.

5. **Top of Shoulder, Back of the Neck, and Temples:** To relieve tension, you should apply the right essential oil, such as PanAway or Peppermint, to these areas.

6. **Wrists, Behind Ears, and Across Forehead:** To boost your mind, you should apply the right essential oil (such as Joy, Citrus Fresh, and Frankincense) to these areas.

7. **Behind the Earlobes, Crown of the Head, and Center of the Head between the Eyebrows**: Topical application to these areas is perfect for night time oils, such as Cedarwood, Stress Away, and Lavender.

8. **General Skin:** To achieve skin moisturization using the right blend of oil, you can apply the oil recipe/blend generally on your skin.

9. **On Scars:** Oils, such as Lavender and Frankincense, are neat and good for bruises and scars.

10.**Sore Muscles:** Massage, then use appropriate oil.

Topical application means applying the oils straight onto the skin surface according to label directions. The oils can be applied on the soles of the feet, ears, hands, along the spine, back, or on the area of concern. It is recommended that oils be diluted before usage with children. Most often, essential oils are applied before a massage, after a massage, or during a massage on any part of the body, from the head to the feet. Apart from the skin massages, one of the most effective and safest places of applying essential oils is the soles or bottom of the feet. This method is particularly recommended for people with skin sensitivities, allergies and children, and is the best place to conduct "oil sensitivity" testing.

TOPICAL APPLICATION TECHNIQUES

1. **Reflex Points and "Vita Flex" Technique:** The technique involves stimulating the nerve

pathways leading to different internal body systems. It is an effective technique for achieving therapeutic effects throughout the body, but it can also effectively target specific support areas of the body. Reflex points are located on both the hands, ears, and feet, and when stimulated, the essential oils are quickly absorbed and distributed to target sites, resulting in rapid support. The feet are the most ideal location for topical application of essential oils through reflexes because they allow the oils to reach the bloodstream quickly and are tough enough to reduce the likelihood of irritation and other adverse reactions. The feet can also be covered easily especially if you do not like the aroma of the oil or if you are using the oil with a child and do not want the child to touch the oil. Besides, the reflex points of the hand and feet are connected directly to different organs of the body, and you can easily use visual reflexology guides to identify the points of applying the oils. For treating specific conditions, the Vita Flex Technique is recommended.

2. **Raindrop Technique:** This technique is used to deliver essential oils for supporting the immune system, relieving anxiety and stress, and promoting balance and relaxation. The raindrop technique is a relatively easy method that blends essential oils with massage in order to support the body in a variety of ways.

3. **Massaging:** Essential oil massages are quite enjoyable and effective as techniques for applying the oils to muscles, joints, and tissues. When massaging the body, do not apply excessive pressure to sensitive areas, such as the spinal cord, and you must move towards the heart when massaging legs and hands.

4. **Auricular Technique (Physical and Emotional):** This technique involves the application of essential oils to acupressure points (small reflex points) on and around the ears. The technique delivers therapeutic benefits of the essential oils into the body and to emotional centers of the brain, addressing physical and emotional problems. For instance, drops of

Lavender can be massaged on reflex points of the ears to calm a crying child.

5. **Essential Oil Compress:** To achieve deeper penetration of essential oils, creating a compress is recommended. You can do this by rubbing 1-3 drops of essential oils on the location and covering with a comfortably hot or damp towel. The moist towel should then be covered with a dry towel for 10-60 minutes. A warm feeling will be experienced, but if the feeling becomes uncomfortable, you should apply vegetable (carrier) oil to the location. Oils for muscles and joints are effectively applied, using cold or hot compresses.

6. **Essential Oil Baths:** Oils do not usually mix with water and must be properly dispersed to avoid skin irritation. To achieve this, 5-7 drops of essential oil should be added to 1 cup of baking salt, Epsom salt, or bath gel base. Then, disperse the mixture under running water, as the bath tub fills or sprinkle the mixture into the water after the tub is full. Use your hand to diffuse the essential oil around the bath water.

7. **Essential Oil Foot Bath:** Foot baths are invaluable for relaxation after being extremely stressed, overworked, or tired. Add warm water in a basin or tub and then add 5-10 drops of the essential oil, and then soak your feet for 15-30 minutes.

8. **Directly to the Area of Concern:** Essential oils can be applied directly to the abdomen, chest, back of the neck, energy centers, and other areas of concern after diluting them appropriately.

9. **Personal Care Products:** Essential oils can be applied as personal care products, such as homemade deodorants, or when added to lotions, moisturizers, and skin care regimen.

Finally, during topical applications, you should:

a. Remember that citrus oils and a few other oils are photosensitive. Therefore, you must avoid direct sunlight for at least 12 hours after their topical application. If you use Bergamot, then you must avoid sunlight for up to 3 days. In fact, it is advisable to apply photosensitive essential oils in the evening or to areas of the body that will not be exposed to the sun.

b. Remember that you are unique and will react differently to essential oils. Therefore, if you have sensitive skin or are prone to skin reactions, then you must test essential oils first and dilute them well before usage.

c. Use a layering technique when applying two or more oils. Layering means applying one, waiting for 5-30 minutes, and then applying the next essential oil. Do not try mixing oils, if you are not sure of how to do it.

d. When using essential oils, it is important to remember that the following oils are skin irritants and must be used cautiously: cinnamon leaf, basil, allspice, peppermint, Melissa, wintergreen, sweet fennel, cinnamon bark, lemon, fir needle, clove bud, and tea tree.

II. INHALATION OF ESSENTIAL OILS (AROMATIC APPLICATION)

The olfactory system is made up of physical organs and the cells relating/contributing to the sense of smell. Inhalation refers to the process by which volatile essential oil molecules become vapor and are passed rapidly through the cilia lining of the nasal passage to the olfactory nerve for transportation to the olfactory bulb and then into the brain. Apart from conveying the essence to the brain, inhalation allows airborne essential oil molecules to interact with olfactory organs.

For instance, during inhalation, the odor molecules interact with receptor sites of the limbic system, which controls blood pressure, heart rate, memory, stress levels, breathing, and hormone balance. Once in the brain, the essential oil molecules may also enter the hypothalamus, ANS, or pituitary gland. Likewise, the molecules may pass into the cerebral cortex of the brain, stimulating learning, memory, and emotional responses. Equally, there are several blood vessels in the alveoli of the lungs and nasal mucosa, which help to absorb the oils and to distribute them to the rest of the body.

Essential oils can be inhaled after diffusing them in special essential oil diffusers, humidifiers, scent pods, boiling pot of water, or by simply smelling the oil directly from the bottle. The effectiveness of different delivery methods vary from method to method, with the essential oil diffuser being the most expensive but most effective inhalation method. The oils can either be inhaled through the mouth or nose, as long as they can be strongly diffused to produce the desired effects through the nose or mouth. Moreover, there are several essential oils that can give therapeutic effects when delivered aromatically. For example, Lavender can be inhaled to reduce stress; Wild Orange can be inhaled to improve mood; Peppermint can be inhaled to boost energy and improve focus; Frankincense can be inhaled for enhanced spiritual enhancement; Eucalyptus can be inhaled to reduce coughing; and Melaleuca can be used to cleanse air.

BENEFITS OF AROMATIC APPLICATION OF ESSENTIAL OILS

a. Inhalation of essential oils can nurture the respiratory system, including nasal sinuses.

b. This process protects against airborne threats and increases the quality of indoor air.

c. This process improves mood and hormonal balance and reduces tension, among other effects.

d. Chemical components of the oils access the bloodstream and promote well-being in a number of ways, including killing micro-organisms and boosting immunity.

Aromatic application techniques can help to:

a. Purify air while inhaling healthy immunity-supporting fragrance. For instance, placing a diffuser of essential oils in your family rooms, bathrooms, bedrooms, or anywhere in your home will help to clean and boost the quality of indoor air.

b. Deter insects. For instance, diffusing Purification Oil will eliminate and deter insects in your home.

c. Elicit a peaceful and sound night sleep. For example, if you want to wake up well-rested, you can diffuse Lavender Oil in your bedroom at night to help relax your mind and give you a peaceful sleep.

d. Provide respiratory support. If you or your family members need support for nasal passages, lungs, sinus, or general respiratory support, essential oils, such as the R.C. Blend, can be invaluable.

e. Boost immune support. Essential oils, such as Thieves, will boost your immunity if diffused in your bedroom or home at night.

f. Create perfume. A number of essential oils, including Sensation and Joy (for women) and Idaho Balsam Fir (for men), can offer nourishing all-day odor when worn as perfumes.

INHALATION TECHNIQUES FOR ESSENTIAL OILS (AROMATIC APPLICATION TECHNIQUES)

1. **Direct Inhalation:** The technique involves either holding the bottle of essential oil a few inches from the nose and then breathing in the aroma or adding 1-2 drops of the oil into your hand and cupping the hand over the nose and mouth. Direct inhalation is a good technique for calming or grounding oils, relieving emotional stress, creating supportive therapy for relieving respiratory congestion, and exerting positive effects on the nervous system. Some oils, such as Cinnamon and Oregano, must be diluted before direct inhalation.

2. **Indirect Inhalation:** The technique involves adding a few drops of the essential oil to a handkerchief, small piece of fabric, pillow case, shirt collar, cotton ball, or other items in order to inhale the scent gradually. For example, if you want to enjoy deeper sleep, then you can add Vetiver to any of the mentioned items and put the item next to your bed.

3. **Cold Air Humidifier:** Using a cold air humidifier will help to diffuse the oil in air and allow you to inhale the aroma. For example, you can use a humidifier when purifying indoor air. Nevertheless, remember that essential oils can damage plastic components, and you must, therefore, choose a humidifier that is made specifically for essential oils.

4. **Steam Tent and Hot Water Vaporizer:** You can simply heat a pot of water and then add 1-3 drops of oil so that when you cover your head with a towel while leaning over the hot water, you will inhale the steam. For example, you can boost your respiratory health by adding Eucalyptus oil to hot water.

5. **Inhaler Tubes:** Furnished with organic cotton pads which have 100% essential oils, inhaler tubes are used for relieving nausea, uplifting mood, relieving stress, providing hormonal balance, reducing nasal congestion, promoting healthy breathing, and eliciting emotional support.

6. **Fans and Vents:** Like indirect inhalation, essential oils can be added to cloths and placed in vents or in front of fans to release the scent for inhalation. For example, you can calm car motion sickness by placing peppermint or ginger in a car vent/window.

7. **Natural Room Deodorizers:** Essential oils can be used to make natural deodorants. For example, a mixture of ½ cup of alcohol (such as vodka) with ½ cup of distilled water and 20-40 drops of essential oil can be added to a decorative jar with the addition of 10 bamboo skewers to the mixture. The bamboo skewers will soak the aroma and spread the scent throughout the room.

8. **Perfume or Cologne:** Essential oils not only smell good when used as perfumes/cologne but are also healthier and safer than chemical-based antiperspirants. For example, you can simply add 1-2 drops of your preferred oil to your wrist, behind your ears, or add the oil to alcohol and mist your clothing or body with it.

9. **Diffusing:** Good diffusers for essential oils are those that use room temperature (cool) air or ultrasonic vibrations to diffuse the oils into air. This ensures that the oil molecules remain air-bound for many hours without affecting the structure of the molecules through heating. Examples of diffusers for aromatic oils include:

(i) **Using unscented candles (Candle Burners):** Using candles that have lost their scents, place 1-2 drops of the essential oil on the candle and then light the candle. You will benefit remarkably from the therapeutic properties of the scent from the lighted candle. Similarly, you can use essential oil burners (made of clay, stone, terra cotta, or glass) in which a few drops of the chosen oil is diluted in a small bowl and heated above a tea light.

(ii) **Fan Diffusers:** The diffusers are powered by either electricity or batteries and work by blowing a stream of air over a pad or tray of oil. There are several types of fan diffusers that you can buy and use for inhalation.

(iii)**Nebulizers:** Nebulizers work by breaking down essential oil into separate tiny molecules and allowing for easier inhalation of the molecules through the lungs. You only need to add at least 10 drops of the oil into the nebulizer (glass nebulizer) and then turn the diffuser on to allow the room to be filled with the essential oil aroma. Nebulizers are one of the most common methods used by aromatherapists for dispersing essential oils.

(iv).**Clay and Terra Cotta Discs:** If you are looking for a competitively priced asset for enjoying your aromatherapy oils, then the Clay and Terra Cotta Discs are good for you. The discs rely on the sun's energy to disperse the scent. You only need to add a few drops of the oil on the disc, and dispersion will occur through the porous surface of the disc in order to clean and refresh the air inside the room/car. With the discs, you do not need electricity, batteries, or flame because the scent will just permeate the porous material.

(v).**Pocket Inhalers:** Custom-made to fit safely inside the nose in order to deliver aromatherapy scents directly to the nose, the pocket inhalers are a portable way of enjoying the therapeutic benefits of essential oils wherever you go. If you do not care about being less fashionable, then you can achieve the same effect by carrying around a tissue, old altoids tin, or cotton ball in a plastic bag.

(vi).**Plug-In Aromatherapy Scent Balls:** Scent Balls rely on electricity to disperse aromatherapy scents throughout a room. You only need to add 1-2 drops of the essential oil onto the scent pad, switch power on, and enjoy the aroma for many hours.

(vii).**Steam Inhalers:** Steam inhalers allow you to add a few drops of essential oil to water and then to inhale the aroma.

(viii).**Diffuser Reeds:** Bamboo reeds can be inserted into slender-necked vases containing essential oils so they can soak up the essence of the essential oil mixture and deliver/diffuse the scent into the room.

(ix).**Car Aromatherapy Diffusers:** These are auto aromatherapy diffusers that are plugged into car cigarette lighters and attached to bottles of essential oils in order to fill the car with aroma. The scent is changed by changing the scent pad or the bottle attached to the diffuser.

(x).**Lightbulb Rings:** Diffuser rings can be fixed directly on top of light bulbs before adding 1-2 drops of the essential oil onto the ring. After switching on power, the light bulb will heat up the essential oil and ensure that the scent fill up the room. The diffuser rings can be made of terra cotta, ceramic, or other natural stones.

INTERNAL APPLICATION OF ESSENTIAL OILS (INGESTION)

Essential oils from spices and herbs (such as rosemary, oregano, thyme, and sage) have been used in foods and drinks for many centuries. In quantities, ranging from 0.1-1% of essential oil volume per food weight (v/w), essential oils and their chemical components have been used to reduce lipid oxidation in many foodstuffs and for favorable taste and pleasant odor of beverages and foods. Nevertheless, the use of flavoring substances in food is governed by the desired flavor intensity, leading to the use of low concentrations and very low exposures of the internal systems to the oils.

When it comes to the use of essential oils for therapeutic purposes, it is usually difficult to control the amount of oils used. As a result, ingestion (internal use) of essential oils has been surrounded with controversy. Even though, some people consider internal use as extremely dangerous and should never be considered under any circumstances, others hold the view that the oils can be used internally under all circumstances. The truth falls somewhere in the middle!

But first, what is meant by internal use of essential oils? Internal use means the use of essential oils in any of the following ways:

a. Taking the oils via mouth (orally).

b. Using essential oil suppositories (either rectal or vaginal).

c. Swishing a mouthwash of essential oil in or around the mouth.

d. Utilizing essential oils in various orifices of the body such as ears, eyes, and nose.

DANGERS AND BENEFITS INVOLVED IN INTERNAL APPLICATION

Essential oils are generally so potent that internal usage may cause harm or negative effects, particularly when used in large quantities. For instance, some of the chemical components of essential oils may irritate the gastrointestinal mucosa and mucous membranes, which are usually more sensitive than the skin. Secondly, ingestion of the oils always carries the potential of inducing nausea and vomiting and may also cause unpredictable effects in the bloodstream. Besides, digestive enzymes can break down some constituents of essential oils (such as esters that may be hydrolyzed in the stomach), and when passed to the liver, they can be converted to toxic by-products. Ingestion also carries greater risk of overdose and interaction with medications. In fact, almost all recorded cases of severe poisoning with essential oils have occurred after ingestion of large quantities of essential oil.

Nevertheless, since the problems associated with internal ingestion are usually concentration-dependent, efficient dispersion (dissolution) or dilution of the oils before administration can reduce their potential adverse effects. Likewise, the risks associated with internal use can be reduced when essential oils are prescribed by qualified naturopathic doctors with experience and knowledge in essential oil pharmacology. Moreover, there are several essential oils that have been approved by the FDA as Generally Regarded as Safe (GRAS) for internal use. When such oils are ingested after consulting naturopathic experts, there is little likelihood that they will harm internal systems.

Furthermore, when essential oils are ingested, the healing properties of the oils will fully enter the body, resulting in better efficacy. Hence, when suffering from a serious health disorder or crisis, it may be acceptable to administer the oils internally but in low quantities. And, obviously, internal application must be reserved for serious conditions and must only occur under the guidance of a naturopathic expert.

High Quality Oil for Internal Use

Ingesting high quality and absolutely pure essential oil will ensure that you do not ingest harmful chemicals or components with unpredictable action. And, because of the high risks associated with internal application of essential oils, the oils used must be high quality. To know if essential oil is High Quality, you should find out whether the oil is genuine and 100% natural (not containing synthetic additives), 100% pure (with no addition of a similar essential oil), 100% complete (not re-colored, deterpenated or decolorized), or authentic and produced from the specific species listed in the label. Similarly, the best essential oils for ingestion must come from production facilities focused on aromatic healing, with every batch processed carefully, slowly, and at low temperatures.

To find top quality essential oil, choose a supplier you trust and let your supplier help you find the oil. You must choose a supplier who knows the farmers and companies producing the oils directly and who takes pride in best-distilled oils with great therapeutic value.

FDA Approved Essential Oils for Oral Administration

The following essential oils have been certified as Generally Recognized as Safe for oral administration: Angelica, Basil, Bergamot, Roman Chamomile, German Chamomile, Cinnamon Bark, Citrus Rind, Clary Sage, Clove, Coriander, Dill, Eucalyptus globulus, Frankincense, Galbanum, Geranium, Ginger, Grapefruit, Hyssop, Idaho Blue Spruce, Juniper, Jasmine, Laurus nobilis, Lavender, Lemon, Lemongrass, Lime, Melissa (Lemon balm), Marjoram, Myrrh, Myrtle, Nutmeg, Orange, Oregano, Patchouli, Pepper, Peppermint, Petigrain, Pine, Rosemary, Rose, Savory, Sage, Sandalwood, Spearmint, Spruce, Tarragon, Tangerine, Thyme, Vetiver, Valerian, and Ylang-Ylang. Before using any of the essential oils orally/internally, a knowledgeable health practitioner should be consulted. For oral ingestion, 3-4 drops of the diluted oils should be taken 1-2 times a day, or 3-10 drops should be added in enema/suppository.

Essential Oils Approved by the German Commission E for Internal Usage

a. Fennel

b. Anise

c. Caraway

d. Cinnamon Bark

e. Lavandula flos

f. Eucalyptus

PRECAUTIONS FOR USING ESSENTIAL OILS INTERNALLY

a. Make sure to use GRAS essential oils.

b. Less Is More: Start off conservatively; use a few drops of the oil. Instead of multiple drops, start with one drop.

c. Use high quality and pure oils only.

d. Increase Frequency of Use before Increasing Quantity: The human liver tolerates essential oils in small doses because it breaks down oils more slowly. Therefore, it is wiser to use 1 drop 15-60 minutes apart than using many drops at once.

e. Reserve Internal Application for Extreme Conditions: Since essential oils can be administered by several methods, you should save internal use for when you need it most.

f. Use Common Sense: Essential oils are highly concentrated and potent, and large doses are bad for you. If you have children, store the essential oil bottles away from their reach. Dilute the oils before use.

g. Limit the Number of Daily Drops: The recommended number of drops per day is 10-25 (with 25 being for oils like citruses).

h. Certain Oils Must Be Used with More Caution: For example, oils with high concentration of phenols (like cinnamon, thyme, and oregano) tend to accumulate in the liver, and must be used with great care.

i. Dilute Always: Since the gastrointestinal tract and mucous membranes are more easily irritated than the skin, you should dilute every essential oil before internal use to minimize potential irritation.

j. Some People Should Avoid Ingestion of Essential Oils: For pregnant women, nursing mothers, people with major health conditions, people with compromised immunities, and people with liver problems, it advisable to avoid internal use of the oils unless advised by a naturopathic physician. People with high blood pressure and epileptics should consult their doctors before using the oils internally. Essential oils must never be administered internally to children under six.

TECHNIQUES OF INTERNAL APPLICATION OF ESSENTIAL OILS

a. **Drinking:** Drops of essential oils can be added to water, almond milk, or rice milk for drinking. For example, lemon or peppermint can be added to water and used to boost energy or digestion. However, since most essential oils will not mix with water, you should stir thoroughly so that oil molecules sink into the water. Besides, you should never mix hot oils with non-oil based liquids because strong oils can irritate your gastrointestinal tract and mucous membranes.

b. **Cooking:** A number of essential oils can be cooked or baked. One drop or less of the oil may be enough, but some recipes may require more. Just make sure to start small.

c. **Rectal or Vaginal Insertion:** This method should be used with caution, and you must first find out whether your vagina or rectum is sensitive to the oil. The oil must be diluted properly, and you should work with a naturopathic expert when going this route.

d. **Supplemental:** You can add 1-2 drops of the essential oil to one teaspoonful of honey and take as a supplement, or buy empty veggie capsules for adding the drops of oils you take daily. You may also buy specially-formulated essential oil supplements for boosting energy, digestion, or immunity.

APPLICATION OF ESSENTIAL OILS EXTERNALLY IN YOUR HOUSE OR ENVIRONMENT

There are many ways of using essential oils in or around the home. Here are some ideas.

a. You can add 1-2 drops of Melaleuca to the kitchen sink, when you are washing dishes.

b. You can use Lemon to remove stains and use Lime to remove stickers, gum, and other residues from most surfaces in your home.

c. You can repel ants and other crawling insects from your home using Arborvitae or Peppermint. You only need to place a few drops of the oil on cotton ball and hide around the entrance, behind the fridge, or around the areas where the insects invade.

d. You can add appropriate essential oil to your washing machine to wet clothes before taking to the dryer or mist the fabrics before taking them to the clothes lines for drying.

e. You can use essential oils as natural household cleaners, such as carpet deodorants, sprays, and furniture polish. For instance, you can mix your favorite oil with baking soda (for carpet powder) by vacuuming.

f. You can add essential oils to craft paints, household paint, or children's dough in order to create more pleasant aroma.

g. You can repel mosquitoes and other biting insects, using insect-repelling essential oils.

CHAPTER 4: PRODUCTION OF ESSENTIAL OILS

Essential oils are extracted from plants or plant parts, using different production processes. Ideally, the extraction processes for essential oils must preserve therapeutic benefits and ensure that most of the targeted chemical components of the oils are obtained. It usually takes 150 pounds of lavender, 50 pounds of eucalyptus, 1000 pounds of jasmine, 500 pounds of rosemary, and more than 2000 pounds of rose to generate a single pound of the respective essential oil. And, the price of every essential oil is directly related to the quantity of plant material used in the extraction.

TYPES OF RAW MATERIALS FOR EXTRACTING DIFFERENT ESSENTIAL OILS

Essential oils are obtained from different plant sections. Here are examples of the raw materials for various essential oils.

a. Essential oils extracted from BERRIES: Allspice and Juniper.

b. Essential oils extracted from SEEDS: Anise, Buchu, Celery, Cumin and Nutmeg.

c. Essential oils extracted from LEAVES: Basil, Buchu, Bay Leaf, Cinnamon, Common Sage, Guava, Eucalyptus, Lemon Grass, Melaleuca, Oregano, Patchouli, Peppermint, Pine, Rosemary, Spearmint, Tea Tree, Thyme, Tsuga, and Wintergreen.

d. Essential oils extracted from FLOWERS: Cannabis, Chamomile, Clary Sage, clove, scented Geranium, Hops, Hyssop, Jasmine, Lavender, Manuka, Marjoram, Rose, Orange, and Ylang-ylang.

e. Essential oils extracted from PEEL: Bergamot, Grapefruit, Lemon, Lime, Orange, and Tangerine.

f. Essential oils extracted from the BARK: Cassia, Cinnamon, and Sassafras.

g. Essential oils extracted from WOOD: Camphor, Cedar, Rosewood, Sandalwood, and Agarwood.

h. Essential oils extracted from RHIZOME: Galangal and Ginger.

i. Essential oils extracted from RESIN: Benzoin, Copaiba, Frankincense, and Myrrh.

j. Essential oils extracted from the ROOT: Valerian.

There are 4 major types of extraction processes, namely, distillation, expression, solvent extraction, and Florasols extraction. Of the four, the first two are the most commonly used methods.

DISTILLATION

The most common essential oils (like peppermint, lavender, eucalyptus, and tea tree oil) are extracted by steam distillation. During the process, the raw materials (bark, roots, wood, leaves, flowers, seeds, or peels) are placed into distillation apparatus (an alembic). The distillation apparatus is put over water, and then the water is heated to produce steam, which passes through the plant materials, causing the material to release essential oil in the form of vaporizing volatile compounds. The vaporized essences, together with steam and other substances, flow through a pipe (coil) running through cooling tanks. The vapors condense into liquid (called herbal distillate, hydrolat, hydrosol, or plant water essence), which is separated from the water and collected in the receiving vessel. While most essential oils are distilled in a single process, one important exception is Ylang-Ylang (Cananga odorata), which is extracted using fractional distillation.

EXPRESSION

Also called cold-pressing, expression is used exclusively for citrus oils (similar to extraction of olive oil). Because of the relatively large quantities of oil in citrus peel and the low cost of growing and harvesting raw materials, it is generally cost-effective to extract citrus oils by pressing. In expression, the oil-containing outer layer of the fruit is pressed and then filtered to yield the oil. Lemon or Sweet Orange oils are obtained as by-products of the citrus industry.

SOLVENT EXTRACTION

When extracting chemical components that are easily denatured by the high heat of steam distillation or from flowers with too little volatile oil to undergo extraction, solvent extraction is used. During this process, a hydrophobic solvent, such as supercritical carbon-dioxide or hexane, is added to pounded plant materials. The solvent will then help to extract the oil from the raw material in the form of Concretes, which are a mixture of resins, waxes, the essential oil, and other oil-soluble plant material. To obtain pure essential oil from the Concretes, another solvent, which is more polar in nature (such as Ethyl Alcohol), is added to the Concrete. The alcohol (second solvent) is chilled to -18C/0F for at least 48 hours, causing the lipids and waxes to precipitate. The precipitates are filtered out from the mixture before the alcohol (ethanol) is removed from the remaining mixture by vacuum splurge, evaporation, or both, leaving behind the Absolute.

FLORASOLS EXTRACTION

Florasol is an ozone-friendly refrigerant that was developed to replace Freon. It enables essential oil extraction to occur below room temperature and, therefore, prevents the degradation of the chemical components of the oil by high temperature. Besides, the essential oils obtained by Florasol extraction are pure and contain no-to-little foreign substances. Nevertheless, Florasol is fluoro-chemical (1, 1, 1, 2-

Tetrafluoroethane) and poses danger to the environment because of its global warming potential.

METHODS OF TESTING THE QUALITY OF ESSENTIAL OILS

Essential oils used by aromatherapy practitioners must be pure and high quality. Therefore, when selecting essential oil for your therapeutic needs, it is important to choose oil that is 100% natural and pure. You must also know the country of origin, method of extraction (such as expression or extraction), growing season, the plant part used as raw material, and the reputation of the manufacturing company. Similarly, it is important to buy essential oil that has gone through a battery of tests, confirming its quality and authenticity. Moreover, the results of the tests should be indicated on the label. The four major tests for analyzing the quality of essential oil are specific gravity, gas chromatography/mass spectrometry (GCMS), refractive index, and optical rotation.

a. **Gas Chromatography/Mass Spectrometry (GCMS)**

Gas chromatography is used to separate the individual components of essential oils and to measure the quantity of each component present. It helps to confirm the true botanical identity of an essential oil by comparing the existence and quantities of each constituent. It also helps to screen for missing or non-natural constituents and for constituents that occur in unnaturally high ratios. Mass spectrometry identifies the constituents of essential oils by name and points out those that are commonly added to adulterated or inauthentic oils. The GCMS tests help to answer important questions about the purity and quality of the essential oil.

b. Optical Rotation

Optical rotation is the measure of the direction (left or right) and the degree to which light rays rotate or bend, as they pass through essential oils. Since each type of essential oil is made up of unique constituents that will predictably influence the degree and direction of displacement or rotation of light rays, an inauthentic oil will have a different optical rotation from authentic ones.

c. Specific Gravity (SG)

Specific gravity measures essential oil weight at 25 degree Celsius. Since every essential oil is made up of a unique blend of constituents that will give a predictable weight at a given temperature, an inauthentic essential oil will have a different specific gravity from the SG of the authentic one.

d. Refractive Index

Refractive index measures the speed at which light rays are refracted, when passing through an essential oil. Since every essential oil has unique constituents that will predictably influence the speed and degree of refraction of light, an inauthentic essential oil is identified by the fact that it has a different refractive index from the predictable refractive index of the authentic oil.

CHAPTER 5: GROWING CYCLES AND THERAPEUTIC VALUE OF ESSENTIAL OILS

The physical and emotional therapeutic values of essential oils depend significantly on the plant parts where they are obtained. Typically, the predominant chemical components of plants reside on different plant parts according to the growing phase of the plant (or season of the year) when the plant part is harvested. For instance, the medicinal components of plant roots are usually at their peak or strongest during winter and late fall because the cold seasons compel the plants to draw back their energy into themselves for survival. When spring comes, the medicinal components of the same plants are reaching out and are found in the leaves and stems. Therefore, plant materials for extracting essential oils should be obtained during the right time of the year (phase of plant development) in order to maximize the healing properties of the resulting essential oils.

The growing cycles of essential oil plants usually begin with the seeds, then the roots, followed by leaves, then flowers before producing the fruits (which are the seeds of most plants). The production of the fruits marks the beginning of another cycle as the plants return to the physical world. During different stages of growth, the plants produce chemicals, woods, resins and aromas that have medicinal value.

THERAPEUTIC VALUE OF ESSENTIAL OILS FROM SEEDS

Essential oils obtained from plant seeds (such as coriander oil and fennel oil) are generally regarded as capable of inspiring new experiences in our lives and enabling us to make dramatic changes. Typically, essential oils obtained from seeds have great impact on the growth and development of the body. They improve the structure and function of body organs, such as digestive organs and glands. They also cleanse and support the liver, helping the body to eliminate accumulated toxins and poisons. Similarly, the oils derived from seeds boost creativity and intuition, resulting in better output at the workplace, improved relationship with others, increased self-love and efforts to improve your appearance and surroundings, and more understanding of the world around you.

So when should you use essential oils extracted from seeds? The essential oils are vital when you feel insecure, disillusioned, self-pitying, despondent, overwhelmed, and worthless because they can revive your energy and stability and change your view of life. You should also try these oils, if you have been jumping from one job to another or from project to project without being satisfied. Examples of seed essential oils to consider are Nutmeg, Parsley, Manuka, Fenugreek, Fennel, Cumin, Coriander, Caraway, Celery Seed, Carrot Seed, Anise, Anethi, and Ajowan.

THERAPEUTIC VALUE OF ESSENTIAL OILS EXTRACTED FROM FRUITS

The fruits of plants usually contain seeds and typically represent the capacity to have sufficient energy for a long time. In fact, while there are a variety of plants with different kinds of fruits, the essential oils extracted from fruits seem to share the same ability to nourish the organs and glands of the body. Some fruit essential oils will nourish the nervous system, some the skin, some the circulatory system; while others will nourish the glands and eliminate glandular deficiencies. Besides, fruit-extracted essential oils help us to feel friendly, kind-hearted, supportive of others, dependable, joyful, passionate and diligent, and enable us to feel connected and satisfied with ourselves.

These essential oils should be used by individuals who are feeling indecisive, contradictory, unreasonably defensive, clingy, oversensitive and anxious, hesitant and over-cautious, sarcastic, impatient, spiteful and inferior. The essential oils can also help people who cannot stick to their jobs or projects because of indecision or because they are easily and frequently feeling hurt by people or events. Examples of fruit essential oils are Anise, Allspice, Bergamot, Black Pepper, Clove, Green Pepper, Lemon, Lime, Mandarin, Orange, Vanilla, Tangerine, Clementine, Cinnamon Berry, Juniper Berry, Chaste Tree, Grapefruit, Zanthoxylum, Litsea Cubeba, and Suganhda Kokila.

THERAPEUTIC VALUE OF ESSENTIAL OILS EXTRACTED FROM ROOTS

Essentials oils extracted from the roots have grounding, peaceful energy and nourishing and strengthening qualities. The oils are potent stimulants of fundamental body functions (such as digestion and nerves) and are commonly recommended for anemia and other medical conditions associated with poor nutrient absorption. Besides, these essential oils enable us to enjoy harmony in our lives and to be firmly grounded in ourselves so that we can be good-natured but firm. By promoting internal strength, the oils enable us to trust ourselves and others, to be observant, loyal, reliable, teachable and humble, to be self-confident yet not overbearing, and to establish successful relationships with a huge variety of people.

Root essential oils are invaluable to individuals who are often disorganized, moody, apathetic, depressed, obstinate, confused in their thinking, neglectful of the people left under their care, or overly emotional. The essential oils are also useful during pregnancy because they promote nutrient absorption, nervous function, energy and emotional balance, eliminating the mood swings, and other problems associated with early stages of pregnancy and nursing. Commonly used root essential oils are Vetiver, Valerian, Spikenard, Ginger, Garlic, Calamus, Angelica, and Turmeric.

THERAPEUTIC VALUE OF ESSENTIAL OILS EXTRACTED FROM LEAVES

Essential oils extracted from plant leaves provide amazing toning (or cleansing) effects on the body, promote knowledge acquisition processes, and have unique affinity to the respiratory system. The oils not only help us to have better mental focus, energy, and confidence to carry our ideas to fruition, but also boost our creative thinking. People who use leaf essential oils have a tendency to avoid conflict and aggression.

Leaf essential oils should be used by people who are feeling paranoid, hostile, cynical, scornful, exhausted, or overwhelmed. Students can also use the essential oils to promote their understanding of complex subjects and to help them keep the whole picture in mind, even as they specialize in sub-disciplines. The oils are also good for people who are feeling exhausted or resentful of the demands of keeping their families or friends.

Common leaf essential oils are Allspice, Basil, Bay, Anthopogon, Blue Tansy, Camphor, Cinnamon, Clary Sage, Fir, Eucalyptus, Davana, Cypress, Citronella, Cassia, Cajuput, Birch, Wintergreen, Violet Leaf, Pine, Tarragon, Tea Tree, Spruce, Spearmint, sage, rosemary, Rose Geranium, Ravensara, Peppermint, Patchouli, Palmarosa, Oregano, Niaouli, Myrtle, Melissa, Marjoram, Ledum, Kanuka, Ginger Grass, Geranium, and Galbanum.

THERAPEUTIC VALUE OF ESSENTIAL OILS EXTRACTED FROM FLORALS

While only small quantities of essential oils are found in flowers, the fragrances of such oils are usually more intense and may be exhilarating or mildly intoxicating. Floral essential oils are obtained from petals of trees, flowers and shrubs, and are useful in relieving many physical ailments, pain, nervous tension, and emotional stress. The essential oils are also good for problems of the female reproductive cycles. Since humans almost naturally feel the need to be complemented and admired by others, floral energy can help us to replace our feelings of inadequacy with a burst of confidence, enthusiasm, passion, love, dynamism, and energy, enabling us to live our lives happily regardless of our core personalities or what others think of us.

Floral essential oils should be used by individuals who are becoming overly manipulative, insensitive, have difficulties loving and sharing with others, have shallow values, lie frequently to appear good or achieve goals, envious of status, or power hungry. Common outstanding floral essential oils are Ylang-Ylang, Yarrow, Violet Leaf, Tagette, Rose (Maroc and Otto), Patchouli, Osmanthus, Neroli, Melissa, Lavender, Jasmine, Idaho Tansy, Helichrysum, Goldenrod, Chamomile, Cantip, Blue Tansy, and Anthopogon.

THERAPEUTIC VALUE OF ESSENTIAL OILS EXTRACTED FROM WOOD

Wood essential oils have grounding and centering properties, helping us to be full of confidence in our abilities and to be flexible enough to adapt to changes in our environment. Obtained from the shavings, twigs or chippings of shrubs and trees, wood essential oils treat many physical ailments, especially skin conditions and glandular disharmonies. They are useful for improving heart irregularities, nervous tension, stress and depression, and ability to cope with difficult situations. Wood essential oils also help us to be independent, strong, bold and forthright, standing for justice, and showing compassion to others for their mistakes.

Wood essential oils are useful for people who are dictatorial, unyielding, threatening, and expecting others to accept their opinions and decisions without question. When such people use the oils, they regain the necessary internal harmony and balance, which can help them to live in harmony with others. Common wood essential oils are Cypress, Camphor, Cabreuva, Cedarwood, Galbanum, Pine, Hinoki, Howood,

Cinnamon, Spruce, Sandalwood, Rosewood, and Ravensara.

THERAPEUTIC VALUE OF ESSENTIAL OILS EXTRACTED FROM RESINS/GUMS

Extracted from balsam or resin that exudes from the bark of certain shrubs and trees, resin essential oils have amazing affinity for glandular systems. They boost vital body secretions, improve physical healing (catarrhal conditions, inflamed and pus-filled infections, inflammations and ulcers), and demonstrate cosmetic value (restoring skin elasticity). Resin essential oils also promote deep spirituality, love for high moral values (truth, justice, and purity), and realistic outlook of life.

The essential oils are useful for people who are unforgiving. hypercritical, self-righteous, intolerant, dogmatic, nervous, and depressed. Common resin essential oils are Myrrh, Frankincense, Copaiba Balsam, Benzoin, and Opoponax.

THERAPEUTIC VALUE OF CULINARY SPICES

Although spice essential oils are extremely varied in nature, they are typically high in minerals and are useful in severe infections by resistant bacteria, extreme fatigue, complete collapse, and unusually volatile emotions. The essential oils boost our cellular oxygen levels and make us animated, warm-hearted, dynamic, spontaneous, happy, energetic, self-assured, productive, and practical. They are sedative during times of stress, stimulant during times of low energy, and toning to the body and mind. The oils can help people who are becoming rude, abusive and resentful, demanding, insulting, or who feel they should treat others as servants. The oils are also useful for relieving depression, panic attacks, and hysteria. Common spice essential oils are Anise, Turmeric, Tarragon, Rosemary, Oregano, Nutmeg, Marjoram, Ginger,

Lemongrass, Dill, Cumin, Coriander, Clove, Cinnamon, Cardamom, Caraway, Black Pepper, and Basil.

THERAPEUTIC VALUE OF MEDICINAL HERBS

Essential oils extracted from herbal plants are generally called medicinal herbs. Boasting of high concentrations of nutrients, the oils offer a wide range of benefits to the body and mind. They relieve nutritional deficiencies and promote well-nourished body systems. Common examples of herbal essential oils are Clary Sage, Basil, Geranium, Hyssop, Melissa, Myrtle, Green Yarrow, Blue Yarrow, Thyme (both red and white), Sage, Rosemary, Oregano, Spearmint, and Peppermint.

CHAPTER 6: PRINCIPLES OF DILUTING ESSENTIAL OILS

Essential oils are lipophilic compounds that do not usually mix with water. Therefore, they are usually diluted in organic solvents, such as polyethylene glycol and pure ethanol. Dilution of essential oils is important for two reasons. First, dilution helps to avoid skin reactions, such as irritation, phototoxicity, and sensitization. Secondly, dilution helps to avoid systemic toxicity, such as hepatotoxicity, neurotoxicity, carcinogenicity, and ferotoxicity. While there are instances when experienced aromatherapy practitioners may make exceptions and use essential oils undiluted, it is not advisable to use any essential oil without diluting (not even Lavender) because of the potential of facing dire consequences.

For instance, undiluted essential oil (even if it is just one drop of lavender) can cause permanent sensitization when the oil lands on broken skin. The symptoms of skin sensitization vary from one person to the other but typically occur in the form of a skin allergy, which results in severe and itchy rash.

Extremely severe cases of sensitization may lead to respiratory problems or even to anaphylactic shock. Besides, after you develop sensitization to a given essential oil, you will remain permanently sensitized to it even if you begin to dilute it properly before usage. Furthermore, you may develop sensitization reactions to other essential oils and to products containing these oils. Therefore, it is really not worth it trying to use essential oils undiluted. On the contrary, diluting essential oils will save you money and protect your wellbeing.

Treating Essential Oils with Respect

Essential oils are typically highly concentrated and potent. They deserve to be treated with the same care and respect accorded to medicines. While you should not be afraid of the oils, you should also remember that every therapeutic agent comes with adverse effects when used incorrectly, and essential oils are not exception. And, just like medicines, where less is more; the little quantity of essential oils you use the better. Treating essential oils with respect also means diluting oils before using and avoiding all oils that are more likely to cause sensitization or irritation on your skin.

Besides, respecting the oils means conducting a skin patch test when using any essential oil for the first time.

CORRECT DILUTION OF ESSENTIAL OILS

Essential oils are diluted by adding a drop (drops) of the essential oil into carrier oil. Carrier oils are usually obtained from the fatty portions of plants and act as effective media for absorption of the essential oils into the skin, while helping to spread the essential oil over a larger surface area, resulting in more effect. The carrier oil also keeps the essential oil longer and gentler on the skin. Nevertheless, the carrier oil you select for the dilution should be high quality and should be preferably oil that has been cold-pressed.

The most common carrier oils to essential oils are:

a. **Jojoba Oil:** It is highly penetrative and good for diluting oils to be used for psoriasis, eczema, acne, inflamed skin, and all skin types. It is used as an additive to base oil and must not exceed 10%.

b. **Sweet Almond Oil:** It is ideal for relieving soreness, redness, itching, and inflammation on all skin types; it can be used as base oil (100%).

c. **Avocado Oil:** It can be used for all skin types, but is more useful for dehydrated and dry skin types and for treating eczema. It is used as additive to base oil and must not exceed 10%.

d. **Coconut Oil:** The oil has less oily residue than other carriers and less odor. It can be used for all skin types, but is nicer for dry or damaged skin. It is used 100% as base oil, but MUST never be added to any carrier oil blend.

e. **Grapeseed Oil:** It is good for all skin types and can be used as 100% base oil.

f. **Olive Oil:** It has amazing soothing effect and is good for hair care, rheumatic conditions, and cosmetics. It is used as additive to base oil, not more than 10%.

g. **Pomegranate seed oil:** It is used with all skin types--100%.

h. **Hazelnut oil:** It has slight astringent action and is good for all skin types. It is used 100%.

i. **Kukui Oil:** It is used with all skin types-- additive to base oil (not more than 10%).

j. **Wheat-germ oil:** It demonstrates action against eczema, psoriasis, and prematurely aged skin; it can be used on all skin types but only as additive to base oil (not more than 10%).

k. **Sesame Oil:** It shows action against rheumatic conditions, eczema, psoriasis, and arthritis. It is good for all skin types but used as additive to base oil (not more than 10%).

l. **Apricot Oil:** It is good for all skin types but is more useful on prematurely aging skin, inflamed skin, sensitive, or dry skin. It can be used as base oil (100%).

m. **Macadamia Oil:** It is used with all skin types-- additive to base oil (not more than 10%).

n. **Evening Primrose Oil:** It helps to prevent premature aging of the skin and is good for blends used to treat multiple sclerosis, menopausal problems, and heart disease. It is excellent in the treatment of psoriasis and eczema. It is used as additive to base oil (no more than 10%).

o. **Carrot Oil:** It is good for premature aging, itching, dryness, psoriasis, and eczema. It rejuvenates the skin and reduces scarring but must Never be used undiluted. It is used as additive to base oil. It must not exceed 10%.

p. **Borage Oil:** It is good for all skin types but is particularly useful for multiple sclerosis, menopausal problems, heart disease, psoriasis and eczema, and prematurely aged skin. It regenerates and stimulates the skin. It is used as additive to base oil and must not exceed 10%.

q. **Corn Oil:** It is used with all skin types (100%).

r. **Peanut Oil:** It is used with all skin types (100%).

s. **Safflower Oil:** It is used with all skin types (100%).

t. **Sunflower oil:** It is used with all skin types (100%).

u. **Soy Bean Oil:** It is used with all skin types (100%).

To keep carrier oils fresh and useful, you should store them away from light and heat. In fact, you should store you carrier oils, essential oils, and blends in the refrigerator to extend their shelf life. Moreover, you should add 10% Jojoba Oil to your carrier oils and blends to extend their shelf life. Similarly, adding Vitamin E (an excellent anti-oxidant) to your carrier oils and oil blends will extend their shelf life.

DILUTION RATIOS

The extent of diluting essential oils depends on the issue to be addressed. Here are the basic dilution guidelines for various circumstances:

a. 0.25% Dilution (1 drop of essential oil into 4 teaspoonfuls of carrier oil): This is a dilution guideline for children between 6 months and 6 years. You must remember that essential oils are only administered to children when absolutely necessary. Try avoiding essential oil application in children under 2 years and to use herbs/hydrosols instead.

b. 1% Dilution (1 drop of essential oil into 1 teaspoonful of carrier oil or 5-6 drops of essential oil per ounce of carrier oil): This dilution is recommended for children above 6 years, the elderly, pregnant women, individuals with sensitive skin, persons with compromised immunity, and persons with serious health conditions. This is also the best dilution to use when massaging a large area of the body with essential oil.

c. 2% Dilution (2 drops of essential oil into 1 teaspoonful of carrier oil; or 10-12 drops of essential oil per ounce of carrier oil): This dilution is ideal for most (healthy) adults, most health conditions, and daily skin care.

d. 3% Dilution (3 drops of essential oil into 1 teaspoonful of carrier oil; 15-18 drops of essential oil per ounce of carrier oil): This is a short-term dilution that is used for temporary health conditions, such as respiratory congestion and muscle injury. Up to 10% dilution may be fine, depending on the person's age, health condition, health concern, and type of oil being used.

e. 25% Dilution (25 drops of essential oil into 1 teaspoonful of carrier oil; 125-150 drops of essential oil into 1 ounce of carrier oil): This rare dilution is used only when warranted. It is used for bad bruising, severe pain, and muscle cramps.

In order to dilute essential oils properly, you should know the following measurement equivalents:

a. 1 ounce = 30 ml = 6 tsp = 600 drops

b. 5/6 ounce = 25 ml = 5 tsp = 500 drops

c. 2/3 ounce = 20 ml = 4 tsp = 400 drops

d. ½ ounce =15 ml = 3 tsp = 300 drops

e. 1/3 ounce = 10 ml = 2 tsp = 200 drops

f. 1/6 ounce = 5 ml =1 tsp = 100 drops

g. 1 ml of essential oil = 900 mg of essential oil

h. 1 drop of essential oil = 30 mg of essential oil

RECOMMENDED DILUTION FOR DIFFERENT APPLICATION METHODS

(a).Dilution For Massage/Body Oil

Essential oils are usually diluted with one or more vegetable oils before usage in body massage. The massages are targeted at relieving stress, anxiety, headaches, migraines, insomnia, chronic pain, acute pain, arthritis, rheumatism, chronic muscle and joint pain, and enhancing immunity. Body massage with diluted essential oils also reduces inflammation, helps during pregnancy and labor, relieves muscle spasms, soothes the nervous system, and aids the treatment of sprains and other movement injuries.

-For massaging children, the recommended dilution is 0.5% to 1% (or 3-6 drops of essential oil into one ounce of carrier oil).

-For massaging adults, the recommended dilution is 2% to 10% (15-60 drops of essential oil into one ounce of carrier oil), depending on age, heath status, and concern being treated.

a) Facial Lotions, Creams and Oils

After buying unscented facial creams, lotions or oils, you can add the right essential oil to them. Similarly, you can create homemade facial oil, using a variety of vegetable oils and then adding your desired aroma using the right essential oils. Addition of essential oils to facial creams or lotions can help to boost wound healing, slow down aging, boost skin tone, reduce scars, improve facial appearance, balance sebum production, increase local circulation, boost skin hydration, soften and soothe the skin, aid skin detoxification process, enhance immunity, and address emotional issues.

-For adults with sensitive skin, the recommended dilution is 0.5%-1% (3-6 drops of essential oil into one ounce of carrier oil).

-For adults with normal healthy skin, the recommended dilution is 1%-2.5% (6-15 drops of essential oil into 1 ounce of carrier oil).

b) Essential Oil Baths

Essential oil baths are used to reduce stress and anxiety, alleviate muscle tension and pains, soothe mental and physical fatigue, stimulate blood circulation, aid detoxification, reduce pain and stiffness, enhance lymph circulation, improve skin health and tone, and boost local circulation. To prepare an essential oil bath, it is recommended that you add 2-12 drops of essential oil to 1 teaspoonful of whole milk, honey or vegetable oil, and then add the mixture to the bath after you are inside the bath. Some essential oils can sting the body, so you must add NOT more than 2 drops of the following STINGING oils to your bath: orange, lemon, aniseed, camphor, grapefruit, eucalyptus, ginger, juniper, clove, peppermint, black pepper, savory, sage, thyme, and spearmint.

c) Essential Oil Footbaths

Essential oil footbaths are invaluable for individuals who are immobile or too fragile to use other application methods. The footbaths are effective in relieving stress. The recommended dilution is 2-12 drops of essential oil into 1 teaspoonful of carrier oil before adding the mixture to a bowl of warm water and soaking the feet in the water for around 20 minutes.

d) Localized Massage

Essential oils can be applied to small areas, such as stiff joints, cramps and sprains. Since the area to be covered with the oil requires fast action, the dilution used is typically lower than that of facial or body massages but must still offer a safe dosage. The recommended dilution for otherwise healthy adults is 5%-25%, depending on the condition and the area being massaged.

e) Water Compresses

Water compresses are used for situations requiring fast action, such as bruises, cuts, sprains, sunburn, rashes, insect bites, inflammation, and skin infection. The recommended dilution is 2-12 drops of essential oil into 100 ml of hot or cold water. After adding the oil to water, agitate the water, and soak a piece of sterile gauze. Wring out the gauze and apply to the area of concern.

f) Essential Oil Sprays

Sprays of essential oils are made by adding water into spray bottle and then adding 8-10 drops of the specific oil into 300 ml of water. Since oil does not mix with water, you must shake the bottle vigorously before using the spray. Do not get the spray into your eyes or onto painted surfaces.

g) Steam Inhalation

Inhaling essential oils, such as eucalyptus, thyme, lemon or tea tree, can help decongest upper respiratory tract, enhance respiratory function, and treat sinus infections. Add 3-9 drops of the essential oil into boiling water then cover your head with a towel and bend over the steam to breathe the aroma. Keep your eyes closed.

The table below is a summary of popular dilutions for different application methods:

Application	No. of drops of essential oil	Amount of carrier
Massage oil/Lotion	50-60	4 ounces of carrier oil
Topical application	50-60	1 ounce of carrier oil
Ointment	50-60	2 ounces of carrier oil
Footbath	8-10	1 bowl of water
Bath	5-15	Tub full of water
Compress	5	8 ounces of water
Facial oil	6-8	1/3 ounce of carrier oil
Facial mask	2-3	1 teaspoonful of clay
Facial Sauna	2-5	1 bowl of warm water

Body mist	10-20	4 ounces of water
Hair oil	10-20	1 ounce of oil
Cleanser	10-15	4 ounces of oil
Room Spray	20-30	4 ounces of oil
Washing machine	10-20	1 load
Light-Bulb Ring/Auto Vent	1-3	-
Vacuum Cleaner	5-10	-
Artificial holiday Tree	10-15	-

Always remember that essential oils are highly concentrated, and a single drop can go a long way. Therefore, you should dilute the oils properly to avoid high concentrations that may cause skin sensitization, irritation, and other adverse effects. Moreover, you must always use pure high-quality essential oils from a trusted source.

CHAPTER 7: SPECIFIC PROPERTIES AND USES OF ESSENTIAL OILS

There are several essential oils with different properties, therapeutic value, uses and contraindications. When selecting any essential oil for whatever usage, it is prudent to know the properties of the oil and make certain that it is appropriate for the intended use. For instance, Lavender has the capacity to boost the alpha waves of the brain (back of the head), relax the mind, and boost quality of sleep. Jasmine increases the beta waves of your brain (front of the head), making you more mentally alert. Lemon and Eucalyptus fragrances improve mental alertness and have been used in banks and offices to keep staffs alert and reduce potential staff mistakes by up to 54%. Likewise, Rosemary and Lavender are used in customer service areas to calm down customers who are in long waiting lines. Equally, many different essential oils are used to relieve stress, anxiety, muscular and rheumatic pain, women problems (like menopausal complaints, PMS, and postnatal depression), digestive disorders, psychosomatic induced problems, and other concerns.

Top 20 Uses of Essential Oils

1. Air Freshener: A few drops of essential oil are added to a spray bottle and sprayed to improve indoor air quality.

2. Headache Relief: Rub 1 drop of diluted Lavender on your temple.

3. Deterring Ants: Add 2-4 drops of peppermint along the door/window frame where the ants are seen regularly.

4. Freshening Shoes: Place a cotton ball soaked in a few drops of lemon/geranium oil into your shoes and leave in the shoes overnight.

5. Wound Healing: Apply 1-4 drops of diluted lavender to cuts, scratches, scrapes, or bruises to promote healing.

6. Boosting Concentration: Use Rosemary to promote memory and alertness during long car

trips, reading, studying, or preparation for exams.

7. Firewood Aroma: Add 2-4 drops of myrrh or frankincense to dried firewood log and allow the log to soak up the oil before adding the log to fire.

8. Boosting the fragrance and ambience of your room: Add 2-4 drops of your preferred essential oil to a light bulb ring or radiator fragrancer.

9. Reviving Pot Pourri: Add a few drops of your favorite oil to the Pot Pourri.

10. Candle Enhancement: Add 1-2 drops of essential oil to the candle before lighting.

11. Fragrancing Kitchen Drawers and Cupboards: Add a few drops of your favorite essential oil to a cotton ball and then place it in an inconspicuous corner.

12. Boosting the quality of Sleep: Add a few drops of Neroli, Lavender, or Roman Chamomile to your pillow before you retire to bed.

13. Cooling and Protective Baths: Add 5 drops of eucalyptus oil to 1 teaspoonful of vegetable oil, mild foam or milk and then add the mixture to the bath to enjoy cooling baths during the summer and protective baths in the winter.

14. Promoting Healthy Hair: Add 1-2 drops of rosemary to your hair before brushing.

15. Achieving Radiant Skin: Add 1-2 drops of myrrh or geranium to your facial moisturizer.

16. Improve Aroma of Clothes: Add 1-2 drops of your favorite essential oil to a small piece of cloth and place the cloth into the clothes dryer to dry.

17. Treating Viral Illnesses: Add a few drops of lemon and thyme to your diffuser.

18. Adding Scent to your Fridge/Freezer/Oven: Add 1-2 drops of any citrus essential oil to the final rinsing water when cleaning your freezer, oven, or fridge.

19. Stimulating your senses: Add a few drops of grapefruit to your diffuser.

20. Improving workplace productivity: Add a few drops of a blend of grapefruit, lavender, and lemon to the workplace diffuser.

Here is a description of the properties and uses of the most common essential oils:

LAVENDER

Lavender (Lavendula Vera Officinalis) has analgesic, antimicrobial, antidepressant, anticonvulsive, antiseptic, anti-rheumatic, antispasmodic, carminative, antitoxic, deodorant, diuretic, stimulant, sedative, vulnerary, tonic, nervine, cholagogue, cicatrisant, choleretic, cytophylactic, cordial, rubefacient, and insecticide properties. It has a sweet, floral and balsamic aroma and combines well with many essential oils, including clary sage, rosemary, pine, citrus, and patchouli. Lavender oil provides one of the most versatile therapeutic essences. The oil is excellent in first aid, as it soothes bruises, cuts, and insect bites well. It is effective in nervous system disorders, such as headaches, depression, migraine, insomnia, hypertension, nervous tension, PMT, vertigo, sciatica, shock, and stress-related conditions.

Lavender is also useful in treating skin conditions such as acne, abscesses, boils, dandruff, earache, inflammations, eczema, dermatitis, insect stings and bites, bruises, burns, allergies, athlete's foot, scabies, ringworm, sunburn, skin wounds, sores, psoriasis, lice, insect infestations, scars, and spots. Lavender is also used for treating muscular and joint aches and pins, lumbago, sprains, rheumatism, bronchitis, asthma, halitosis, throat infections, laryngitis, whooping cough, colic, abdominal cramps, flatulence, nausea, dyspepsia, cystitis, flu, leucorrhoea, and dysmenorrhea. It is NEAT and can be applied on the skin undiluted, but it is advisable to dilute it before use as a precaution against sensitization reactions. Moreover, Lavender can be used in room sprays, baths, perfumes, colognes, sachets, salves, massage oils, toilet waters, and skin lotions and creams.

1. LAVENDER SPIKE AND LAVANDIN

Lavender spike oil provides a fresh eucalyptus-like aroma that is somewhat like a blend of the aroma of lavender and eucalyptus. The oil blends well with the oils of eucalyptus, rosemary, rosewood, pine, lavender, Petigrain, and Lavandin. It is used an insect repellant, deodorant, disinfectant, air purifier, scent room sprays, and in soaps.

Lavandin is a hybrid resulting from cross-pollination of true lavender and lavender spike. Boasting of a woody spicy-green camphor aroma, Lavandin oil is used in herbaceous colognes, indoor air purification, and clarification and balancing. It blends well with several oils, including citronella, patchouli, pine, thyme, cinnamon leaf, clove, geranium, and cypress.

EUCALYPTUS

Eucalyptus (Eucalyptus Globulus) has analgesic, antiseptic, antispasmodic, anti-rheumatic, balsamic, antiviral, decongestant, deodorant, diuretic, cicatrisant, depurative, febrifuge, expectorant, parasiticide, rubefacient, vermifuge, stimulant, vulnerary, hypoglycemic, and prophylactic properties. It is used for relieving muscular aches and pains, improving blood circulation, relieving asthma, bronchitis, sinusitis, coughs and throat infections, treating sprains, rheumatoid arthritis, flu, colds, measles, leucorrhoea, cystitis, chicken pox and catarrh, and treating nervous system disorders, such as neuralgia, headaches, and debility. Eucalyptus oil is also used to relieve skin disorders, such as blisters, burns, herpes, cuts, wounds, insect bites, skin infections, lice, and as insect repellant. While there are over 300 eucalyptus tree species across the globe, Eucalyptus globulus is the best known species, which has been used for centuries.

LEMON

Lemon (Citrus Limonum) has antiseptic, refreshing, stimulating, antimicrobial, anti-anemic, antiscorbutic, antisclerotic, anti-rheumatic, antitoxic, antispasmodic, bactericidal, astringent, depurative, diuretic, cicatrisant, carminative, diaphoretic, febrifuge, hypotensive, haemostatic, rubefacient, insecticidal, and tonic properties. It stimulates white corpuscles. The scent of lemon is evocative of the fresh ripe peel; while cold-pressed lemon oil is usually more effective than distilled oil. Lemon oil is used for relieving warts, acne, indigestion, depression, cellulitis, arthritis, high blood pressure, obesity, poor blood circulation, nosebleeds, asthma, rheumatism, bronchitis, colds and flu, fever, catarrh, throat infections, dyspepsia, and other infections. Besides, lemon oil is effective in treating anemia, boils, brittle nails, chilblains, cuts, herpes, mouth ulcers, varicose veins, insect bites, spots, greasy skin, and corns. Lemon oil can be added to baths and to massage oils, but it must be diluted properly to avoid skin irritation. Moreover, lemon oil must not be applied on parts that are exposed directly to the sun, as that might result in redness and burning sensation.

2. LEMON EUCALYPTUS, LEMONGRASS AND LIME

Lemon Eucalyptus (Eucalyptus citriodora) gives oil with a fresh, rosy and grass-like aroma, which is similar to the aroma of citronella. It has citronellal as its major chemical component and blends well with eucalyptus globulus oil. It has invigorating and purifying benefits.

Lemongrass oil is obtained by distilling lemongrass, which is a tropical grass that is native to Asia. The aroma of lemongrass oil is powerful, lemony and grassy and is used as insect repellant, vitalizer, and cleanser. Lemongrass oil is added to soaps, detergents, and room sprays.

Lime oil is produced either by distillation or cold-pressing. Distilled lime oil is clear or pale yellow in color and boasts of a perfumy-fruity limeade aroma. On the contrary, cold-pressed lime oil is green to yellow in color and has a rich and fresh lime peel aroma. Lime oil has refreshing and cheering properties, but it may also be applied on the skin after being diluted properly. However, after applying lime oil to the skin, it should not be exposed to sunlight, as this may result in skin irritation.

PEPPERMINT

Peppermint (Mentha Piperita) has refreshing, cooling, digestive, mentally stimulating, anti-inflammatory, antiseptic, analgesic, anti-microbial, astringent, antiviral, cephalic, cordial, cholagogue, carminative, hepatic, expectorant, nervine, vermifuge, antispasmodic, sudorific, and stomachic properties.

Boasting of a powerful, sweet and menthol aroma, peppermint oil is used for treating muscle fatigue, bronchitis, bad breath, indigestion, travel sickness, muscular pain, asthma, palpitations, neuralgia, toothache, sinusitis, skin problems (acne, scabies, ringworm, and dermatitis), spasmodic cough, and digestive problems (colic, dyspepsia, nausea, flatulence, and cramp). Peppermint oil should be thoroughly diluted before use to avoid making the eyes watery and causing the sinuses to tingle.

CLARY SAGE

Clary Sage (Salvia Sclarea) oil has a soothing, antidepressant, aphrodisiacal, warming, antiseptic, anticonvulsive, antiphlogistic, astringent, antispasmodic, aphrodisiac, carminative, bactericidal, digestive, deodorant, cicatrisant, hypotensive, uterine, regulator, nervine, emmenagogue, and tonic properties. Featuring a spicy bittersweet aroma and combining well with many oils, including citrus oils, cardamom, coriander, geranium, Lavandin, sandalwood and cedarwood, Clary Sage oil offers a long-lasting euphoric, visualizing, and centering effect and is an invaluable fixative for other scents. It is used for relieving depression, menstrual problems, high blood pressure, anxiety, asthma, throat infections, muscular pains and aches, cramps, whooping cough, colic, acne, flatulence, dyspepsia, boils, hair loss, dandruff, genitor-urinary tract problems (like dysmenorrhea, amenorrhea, labor pain), inflamed skin conditions, oily hair and skin, wrinkles, ulcers, nervous tension, migraine, headaches, leucorrhoea, impotence, frigidity, and stress-related problems.

GERANIUM (BOURBON)

Geranium (Pelargonium Graveolens) has refreshing, soothing, astringent, antidepressant, anti-inflammatory, anti-hemorrhagic, deodorant, cicatrisant, fungicidal, antiseptic, tonic, stimulant, haemostatic, vulnerary, and diuretic properties. Geranium is one of the most critical perfumery oils and is a regular component of most fragrances. Boasting of a powerful leafy-rose scent with fruity-mint undertones, Geranium oil is used in skin care products, toning and cleansing. Bourbon (Geranium) oil is used for relieving menopausal problems, neuralgia, anxiety, stress, PMT, adrenocortical gland problems, apathy, sore throat, cellulitis, broken capillaries, tonsillitis, breast engorgement, poor circulation, skin complaints (like bruises, acne, burns, cuts, dermatitis, eczema, hemorrhoids, congested skin, broken capillaries, ulcers, wounds, ringworm, mature skin, and oily complexion), mosquito repellant, and lice.

JASMINE

Jasmine (Jasminum Officinale) has analgesic (mild), antiseptic, antidepressant, anti-inflammatory, aphrodisiac, antispasmodic, cicatrisant, carminative, expectorant, parturient, tonic (uterine), sedative, and galactagogue properties. The fragrance of Jasmine is a common component of many perfumes due to its full and rich honey-like sweetness, which offers relaxing, sensual, calming, and romantic effects. Jasmine oil is used for relieving nervous extension, depression, stress-related conditions, coughs, hoarseness, frigidity, dysmenorrhea, laryngitis, labor pains, catarrh, uterine disorders, skin problems (dry skin, sensitive skin, irritated skin, and greasy skin) and muscular sprains, and spasms. Moreover, jasmine is believed to produce a feeling of confidence, optimism and euphoria, and being good for relieving apathy, listlessness, and indifference.

ROSEMARY

Rosemary (Rosmarinus Officinalis) oil has antioxidant, analgesic, antimicrobial, antiseptic, anti-rheumatic, aphrodisiac, antispasmodic, astringent, carminative, digestive, cordial, choleretic, diaphoretic, hepatic, fungicidal, nervine, hypertensive, restorative, parasiticide, stomachic, tonic, rubefacient, hepatobiliary and adrenal cortex systems, and circulatory stimulant properties. Known as a remembrance herb, Rosemary produces an almost colorless essential oil with a fresh and strong camphor aroma. Rosemary oil is used for relieving muscle fatigue, aches and pains, mental fatigue, poor circulation, colds, headaches, debility, neuralgia, nervous tension, mental fatigue, stress-related disorders, asthma, bronchitis, colitis, whooping cough, leucorrhoea, hypotension, hepatic disorders, flatulence, dyspepsia, dysmenorrhea, and hypercholesterolemia. Rosemary oil is also used for treatment of many disorders, such as fluid retention, arteriosclerosis, muscular pains, gout, rheumatism, poor circulation, palpitations, skin conditions (such as eczema, dermatitis, dandruff, acne, and greasy hair). Moreover, Rosemary oil is known for promoting hair growth, repelling insects, and treating scabies, lice, and varicose veins, and stimulating the scalp. The oil is usually a component of citrus colognes, oriental and forest perfumes, eau de cologne, rinses for dark oil, household sprays, soaps, and disinfectants.

SANDALWOOD

Sandalwood (Santalum album) oil has antiseptic, antiphlogistic, antidepressant, astringent, aphrodisiac, bactericidal, antispasmodic, diuretic, carminative, sedative, tonic, insecticidal, fungicidal, and expectorant properties. Endowed with a sweet-woody, balsamic, and warm aroma, which improves with age, Sandalwood blends amazingly with most oils, especially neroli, rose, bergamot, and lavender. The oil is used for relieving insomnia, depression, stress-related complaints, nervous tension, diarrhea, cystitis, bronchitis, nausea, coughs, catarrh, laryngitis, chapped and cracked skin, acne, sore throat, and greasy skin. Sandalwood is a common astringent addition to facial and massage oils, aftershaves, creams and lotions, bath oils, moisturizers, and cleansing agents.

TEA TREE

Tea tree (Melaleuca Alternifolia) oil has antiseptic, antifungal, antiviral, anti-infectious, expectorant, diaphoretic, balsamic, bactericidal, anti-inflammatory, immuno-stimulant, vulnerary, parasiticide, cicatrisant, and fungicidal properties. The oil is spicy, warm, and volatile and is used occasionally to scent aftershaves and colognes. It is also used to relieve pimples, insect bites, athlete's foot, burns, blisters, cold sores, rashes, herpes, abscess, dandruff, mouthwash, acne, cuts, wounds, spots, warts, veruccae, oily skin, infectious illnesses (like chicken pox), vaginitis, cystitis, fever, colds, flu, whooping cough, sinusitis, tuberculosis, catarrh, asthma, and bronchitis. Tea tree oil blends well with nutmeg, rosemary, and Lavandin.

YLANG-YLANG

Ylang-Ylang (Cananga Odorata var genuine) oil has euphoric, anti-infectious, anti-depressant, relaxant, aphrodisiac, antiseptic, hypotensive, anti-seborrheic, tonic, stimulant (circulatory), sedative (nervous), regulator and nervine properties. Produced from freshly-picked flowers of Cananga Tree and endowed with intense, sweet, floral jasmine-like aroma, Ylang-Ylang offers amazing sensual and euphoric benefits. It is used for relieving nervous tension, depression, digestive upsets, palpitations, tachycardia, high blood pressure, and hyperpnoea (abnormally fast breathing). It is also used for treating skin conditions (such as oily skin, irritated skin, insect bites, acne, hair rinse, and hair growth) and nervous system disorders (frigidity, insomnia, impotence, and stress-related disorders).

3. Other Important Essential Oils With Therapeutic Value

a. **ANGELICA ROOT**: Used for dull skin, gout, psoriasis, toxin build-up, water retention, exhaustion, nervousness, and stress.

b. **ANISE**: Used for depression, bronchitis, colds, coughs, flatulence, flu, muscle aches, and rheumatism.

c. **BASIL OIL:** Used for relieving insect bites, insect repellent, muscle aches, rheumatism and sinusitis, fatigue, exhaustion, burnout, memory and concentration, bronchitis, colds, coughs, exhaustion, flatulence, flu, and gout.

d. **BAY OIL**: Used for treating dandruff, hair care, emotional exhaustion and fatigue, neuralgia, oily skin, poor circulation, sprains, and strains.

e. **BENZOIN:** Used for relieving sense of insecurity, arthritis, bronchitis, chapped skin, coughing, and laryngitis.

f. **BAY LAUREL:** Used for boosting confidence, improving mental confusion, and relieving Amenorrhea, colds, flu, loss of appetite, and tonsillitis.

g. **BERGAMOT:** Used for improving anger, anxiety, confidence, depression, stress, fatigue, fear, peace, happiness, insecurity, and loneliness; and for relieving acne, abscesses, anxiety, boils, cold sores, cystitis, halitosis, itching, loss of appetite, oily skin, and psoriasis.

h. **ROSEWOOD (BOISE DE ROSE):** Used for relieving acne, colds, dry skin, dull skin, fever, flu, frigidity, headache, oily skin, scars, sensitive skin, stress, and stretch marks; and for improving depression and emotional imbalance.

i. **CAJEPUT:** Used for relieving asthma, bronchitis, coughs, muscle aches, oily skin, rheumatism, sinusitis, sore throat, and spots; and for improving fatigue and mental confusion.

j. **CARDAMOM:** Used for improving appetite loss of, colic, halitosis, fatigue, stress, shame, and guilt.

k. **CARROT SEED:** Used for relieving eczema, gout, mature skin, toxin build-up, water retention, anxiety, confusion, exhaustion, mood swings, and stress.

l. **CEDARWOOD ATLAS:** Used for relieving acne, arthritis, bronchitis, coughing, cystitis, dandruff and dermatitis; anxiety, fear, insecurity, and stress.

m. **CEDARWOOD:** Used for relieving acne, arthritis, bronchitis, coughs, cystitis, dandruff, dermatitis, insect repellent, stress, anxiety, fear, and insecurity.

n. **GERMAN CHAMOMILE:** Used for treating abscesses, allergies, arthritis, boils, colic, cuts, cystitis, dermatitis, dysmenorrhea, earache, flatulence, hair, headache, inflamed skin, insect bites, insomnia, nausea, neuralgia, rheumatism, sores, sprains, strains, wounds, anger, anxiety, depression, fear, irritability, loneliness, PMS, and stress.

o. **ROMAN CHAMOMILE:** Used for treating abscesses, allergies, arthritis, boils, colic, cuts, cystitis, dermatitis, dysmenorrhea, earache, flatulence, hair, headache, inflamed skin, insect bites, nausea, neuralgia, PMS, rheumatism, sores, sprains, strains, wounds, anger, anxiety, depression, fear, irritability, loneliness, insomnia, and stress.

p. **CINNAMON:** Used for treating constipation, exhaustion, flatulence, lice, low blood pressure, rheumatism, scabies, concentration, and emotional and mental fatigue.

q. **CITRONELLA:** Used for improving excessive perspiration, fatigue, headache, insect repellent, oily skin, mind fog, and tension.

r. **CLOVE BUD:** Used for treating Arthritis, asthma, bronchitis, immune system, rheumatism, sprains, toothache, memory and concentration, fatigue, and depression.

s. **CORIANDER:** Used for treating aches, arthritis, colic, gout, indigestion, nausea, rheumatism, fatigue, and irritation.

t. **CYPRESS:** Used for relieving excessive perspiration, hemorrhoids, oily skin, rheumatism, varicose veins, confidence, grief, memory, and concentration.

u. **ELEMI:** Used for relieving Bronchitis, catarrh, extreme coughing, mature skin, scars, stress, wounds, agitation, and grief.

v. **FENNEL:** Used for relieving bruises, cellulite, flatulence, gums, halitosis, mouth, nausea, obesity, toxin build-up, water retention, fatigue, and emotional imbalance.

w. **FRANKINCENSE:** Used for treating anxiety, depression, fatigue exhaustion and burnout, fear, grief, happiness and peace, insecurity, loneliness, panic and panic attacks and stress; anxiety, asthma, bronchitis, extreme coughing, scars, and stretch marks.

x. **GALBANUM:** Used for treating Immune system abscesses, acne, boils, bronchitis, cuts, lice, mature skin, muscle aches, poor circulation, rheumatism, scars, sores, stretch marks, wounds; emotional rigidity, mood swings, nervousness, and stress.

y. **GINGER:** Used for treating aching muscles, arthritis, nausea, poor circulation, fatigue exhaustion, and burnout.

z. **GRAPEFRUIT:** Used for treating cellulite, dull skin, toxin build-up, water retention, confidence, fear depression, happiness and peace, and stress.

aa. **HALICHRYSUM:** Used for treating abscesses, acne, boils, burns, cuts, dermatitis, eczema, irritated skin, wounds, grief, loneliness, panic and panic attacks, and shock.

bb. **HYSSOP:** Used for treating bruises, coughing, sore throat, respiratory system, concentration, and nervousness.

cc. **JUNIPER BERRY:** Cellulite, gout, hemorrhoids, obesity, rheumatism, toxin build-up, urinary system, agitation, and negative energy.

dd. **LINDEN BLOSSOM:** Used for treating headache, migraine, Acne, dull skin, oily skin, scars, spots, wrinkles, insomnia, stress, and tension.

ee. **MARJORAM:** Used for treating aching muscles, arthritis, cramps, migraine, neuralgia, rheumatism, spasm, sprains, mood swings, PMS symptoms, and stress.

144

ff. **MELISSA:** Used for treating flu, indigestion, herpes, nausea, shingles and cold sores, agitation, anxiety, dementia, and nervous tension.

gg. **MYRRH:** Used for treating amenorrhea, athlete's foot, bronchitis, chapped skin, gums, halitosis, itching, ringworm, emotional imbalance, and creativity.

hh. **MYRTLE:** Used for treating acne, asthma, coughs, hemorrhoids, irritated skin, Addiction and self-destructive behavior, and depression.

ii. **NEROLI:** Used for treating mature skin, oily skin, scars, stretch marks, anxiety, depression, anger, irritability, panic attacks, and stress.

jj. **NIAOULI:** Used for treating acne, bronchitis, colds, coughs, dull skin, oily skin, sore throat, whooping cough, concentration, and mental fog.

kk. **NUTMEG:** Used for treating arthritis, constipation, muscle aches, nausea, neuralgia, poor circulation, rheumatism, mental fatigue, and slow digestion.

ll. **BITTER ORANGE:** Used for treating colds, constipation, dull skin, flatulence, flu, gums, mouth, slow digestion, anger, confidence, depression, fear, and stress.

mm.   **OREGANO:** Used for improving coughs, digestion, respiration, and sense of insecurity.

nn.**PARSLEY:** Used for improving congestion, digestion, diuretic, frigidity, immune system, kidney infections, and stones.

oo.**PATCHOULI:** Used for treating acne, cellulite, chapped skin, dandruff, dermatitis, eczema, mature skin, oily skin, fatigue, frigidity, exhaustion, and stress.

pp.**BLACK PEPPER:** Used for aching muscles, arthritis, detox, constipation, muscle cramps; poor circulation, sluggish digestion, anxiety, concentration, and fatigue.

qq.**PETITGRAIN:** Used for panic, rapid heartbeat, insomnia, and anxiety.

rr. **PINE:** Used for treating colds, congestion, cough; flu, lungs sinusitis, depression, fatigue, and nervous exhaustion.

ss. **ROSE:** Used for treating eczema, mature skin, anger, anxiety, frigidity, depression grief, menopause, happiness and peace, loneliness, panic and panic attacks, and stress.

tt. **SPEARMINT:** Used for treating asthma, exhaustion, flatulence, headache, nausea, scabies, depression, and mental fatigue.

uu.**THYME:** Used for treating arthritis, bronchitis, Candida, cuts, dermatitis, gastritis, laryngitis, concentration, and memory.

vv.**VETIVER:** Used for improving acne, arthritis, muscular aches, oily skin, rheumatism, anger, anxiety, exhaustion, insomnia, fear, grief, insecurity, and stress.

ww.   **VIOLET LEAF:** Used for treating bronchitis, insomnia, liver congestion, sluggish circulation, problem skin, fear, nostalgia, obsession, and shyness.

xx. **YARROW:** Used for treating acne, arthritis, inflammation, hair care; hypertension, insomnia, stress, and tension.

A-TO-Z USES OF ESSENTIAL OILS

A for Anxiety: Add 1-2 drops of diluted Valor Oil to your neck or bottom of your feet. You can also inhale the diluted oil.

B for Brain: To boost your concentration, memory and focus, breathe in a few drops of Peppermint Oil.

C for Colds: Apply 1-3 drops of Thieves oil to upper throat, back, or chest, or to the bottom of your feet and massage the area.

D for Diffuser: Use a diffuser to effectively make essential oil molecules to remain air-borne for inhalation.

E for Ears: Add 1 drop of Helichrysum oil to the outside of your ear and massage properly to treat tinnitus (ringing in the ears).

F for Fatigue: Add 2-4 drops of diluted peppermint to the thyroid region of the neck, temples, or behind the ears 2-3 times daily to relieve fatigue.

G for Gout: Apply 1-3 drops of dilute Frankincense or Juniper oil to the joint and massage gently.

H for Headache: Add a few drops of diluted peppermint on your temples or forehead and massage the area of application.

I for Insect Bite: Apply 1-4 drops of diluted Peppermint, Lavender or Purification blend to the bite are as soon as possible.

J for Joint Pain: Apply 3-5 drops of Peppermint or Wintergreen (diluted 50-50) to the joint and massage gently.

K for Kidneys: Breathe in Lemon essential oil.

L for Lymphatic System: Stimulate and detoxify your lymphatic system by breathing in or diffusing Rosemary or Lemongrass oil.

M for Mosquito Bites: Add 1-2 drops of diluted Lavender or Tea Tree oil to the bite area.

N for NEAT: NEAT refers to oils that can be applied topically undiluted and straight from the bottle. In practice, however, it is advisable to dilute all essential oils before usage, unless recommended otherwise by a naturopathic doctor.

O for Oral Care: Mix a few drops of Spearmint and Peppermint with water and use to brush your teeth or as mouthwash for bad breath and as antiseptic.

P for Pain: Add 2-4 drops of Peppermint oil (diluted 50-50 with water) to the sore muscles and massage gently.

Q for Quick: Essential oils work really quickly. For example, essential oils applied topically will show their effects on the body after 20 minutes or less.

R for Restless Legs: Apply 2-4 drops of diluted Lavender or Chamomile to the legs and massage. You may also diffuse or breathe in the aroma.

S for Stretch Marks: Use 3-6 drops of diluted Lavender or Frankincense two times a day to clear the stretch marks.

T for Sore Throat: Apply a few drops of Eucalyptus oil directly or indirectly to the throat. You may also breathe in the oil, diffuse it, or use steam inhalation method.

U for Underarm Deodorant: Add 10 drops of Lavender to ¼ cup of baking soda; and then apply the blend to your underarms as natural deodorant.

V for Varicose Veins: Rub several drops of Lemon oil on the veins.

W for Wrinkles: Apply 3-4 drops of Frankincense or Lavender oil (diluted 50:50) to the wrinkles. Do not allow the oil to get into your eyes.

X for X-Ray: Use a few drops of Melrose Essential Oil blend (diluted 50:50 with carrier oil) for radiation therapy exposure (protection).

Y for Looking Young: Apply drops of Frankincense oil to your body lotion or oil to help you prevent and reduce wrinkles and make the skin look young and radiant.

Z for Sound Sleep: Add a few drops of Lavender to your pillow to help you achieve relaxing, restful and sound sleep.

A-TO-Z PROPERTIES OF ESSENTIAL OILS

A

ANESTHETIC OILS: Clove, Peppermint, and Cinnamon

ANTI-ALLERGIC OILS: Melissa and Chamomile

ANTI-ASTHMATIC OILS: Cypress, Eucalyptus, Lavender, Frankincense, Roman Chamomile, and Cedarwood

ANTIBIOTIC OILS: Garlic and Tea tree

ANTI-COAGULANT OILS: Geranium

ANTIDEPRESSANT OILS: Bergamot, Benzoin, Lavender, Neroli, Orange, Clary Sage, and Lemongrass

ANTI-MICROBIAL OILS: Thyme, Myrrh, and Tagetes

ANTI-DONTALGIC OILS: Cinnamon, Cajuput, Nutmeg, Pimento, Peppermint, and Cloves

ANTI-NEURALGIC OILS: Cloves, Lemon, Cajuput, and Bay

ANTI-RHEUMATIC OILS: Chamomile, Cajuput, Cypress, Lavender, Lemon, Niaouli, Oregano, Rosemary, Pine, Eucalyptus, Juniper, Thyme, and Hyssop.

ANTI-SCORBUTIC OILS: Ginger, Lemon, and Lime

ANTISEPTIC OILS: Lemon, Lavender, Frankincense, Cloves, Cinnamon, Cedarwood, Camphor, Cajuput, Black Pepper, Bergamot, Basil, sandalwood, Nutmeg, and Rose

ANTISPASMODIC OILS: Aniseed, Bay, Basil, Angelica, Clary Sage, Clove, Bergamot, Camphor, Thyme, Tangerine, Sandalwood, Peppermint, Orange, Neroli, Mandarin, Lavender, and Jasmine

ANTI-SUDORIFIC OILS: Clary Sage

ANTI-VENOMOUS OILS: Thyme and Basil

ANTIVIRAL OILS: Lavender, Eucalyptus, Garlic, Tea Tree, Lime, and Immortelle

ANXIETY OILS: Roman Chamomile, Benzoin, Lavender, Jasmine, Neroli, Sandalwood, and Clary Sage

APERITIF OILS: Bay, Caraway, Cloves, Ginger, Nutmeg, Sage, and Thyme

APHRODISIAC OILS: Clary Sage, Clove, Ginger, Jasmine, Nutmeg, Pimento, Rosewood, Angelica,

154

Aniseed, Basil, Black Pepper, Cinnamon, Sandalwood, Thyme, Vertivert, and Ylang-Ylang

ASTRINGENT OILS: Immortelle, Juniper, Lemon, Lime, Myrrh, Peppermint, Rose, Rosemary, Sandalwood, Yarrow, Bay, Benzoin, Cedarwood, Cypress, Frankincense, Geranium, and Hyssop

B

BACTERICIDE OILS: Lemon, Lemongrass, Lime, Myrrh, Neroli, Rose, Rosewood, Tea Tree, Basil, Garlic, Immortelle, and Lavender

BALSAMIC OILS: Myrrh, Niaouli, Pine, Tea Tree, Cajuput, Clary Sage, and Eucalyptus

BECHIC OILS: Oregano, thyme, Sandalwood, Hyssop, and Ginger

C

CARDIAC OILS: Cinnamon, Hyssop, Nutmeg, Thyme, Aniseed, Black Pepper, and Camphor

CARMINATIVE OILS: Carrot Seed, Cinnamon, Cloves, Ginger, Hyssop, Juniper, Lemon, Lemongrass,

Pimento, Rosemary, Spearmint, Thyme, Melissa, Nutmeg, Orange, Oregano, Parsley, Peppermint, Angelica, Aniseed, Basil, Bergamot, and Black Pepper

CHOLAGOGUE OILS: Peppermint, Rosemary, Rosewood, Bay, Hyssop, and Marjoram

CICATRISANT OILS: Frankincense, Geranium, Hyssop, Juniper, Lavender, Rosemary, Tea Tree, Bergamot, Cajuput, Clove, Cypress, and Eucalyptus

CORDIAL OILS: Lavender, Marjoram, Melissa, Neroli, Peppermint, Benzoin, Bergamot, Rosemary, and Tea Tree

CONCENTRATION OILS: Basil, Black Pepper, and Ginger

CYTOPHYLACTIC OILS: Frankincense, Geranium, Immortelle, Lavender, Carrot Seed, Mandarin, Neroli, and Rose

D

DECONGESTANT OILS: Lavender, Niaouli, Peppermint, Pine, Cajuput, Eucalyptus, and Garlic

DEODORANT OILS: Geranium, Lavender, Lemongrass, Myrrh, Benzoin, Bergamot, Citronella, Clary Sage, Coriander, Cypress, Pine, and Rosewood

DEPURATIVE OILS: Coriander, Eucalyptus, Juniper, Lemon, Rose, Caraway, and Carrot Seed

DETOXIFICATION OILS: Lemon, Orange, Rosemary, Cedarwood, and Grapefruit

DIGESTIVE OILS: Coriander, Ginger, Lemon, Lemongrass, Black Pepper, and Peppermint

DISINFECTANT OILS: Juniper, Lime, Myrrh, Pine, Caraway, and Clove

DIURETIC OILS: Carrot Seed, Cedarwood, Cypress, Eucalyptus, Hyssop, Juniper, Bay, Benzoin, Black Pepper, Lavender, Pine, Rose, Rosemary, Sandalwood, Violet, Lemon, Lemongrass, and Parsley

E

ENERGY OILS: Lemon, Orange, Rosemary, Basil, and Grapefruit

EXHAUSTION OILS: Frankincense, Grapefruit, Lemon, Mandarin, Ylang-Ylang, Black Pepper, and Clary Sage

EXPECTORANT OILS: Bergamot, Cajuput, Cedarwood, Garlic, Peppermint, Sandalwood, Thyme, Angelica, Basil, Hyssop, Myrrh, Parsley, and Pine

FEET (SWEATY) OILS: Cypress, Clary Sage, Geranium, and Peppermint

FEVER OILS: Chamomile, Eucalyptus, Ginger, Lemon, Melissa, Bergamot, and Black Pepper

FLATULENCE OILS: Coriander, and Peppermint

G

GOUT OILS: Juniper, Geranium, and Peppermint

GUM INFECTION OILS: Myrrh, Peppermint, and Tea Tree

H

HANGOVER OILS: Grapefruit, Juniper, Pine, Rosemary, and Cypress

HAY FEVER OILS: Lavender, German Chamomile, Eucalyptus, and Melissa

HYPERTENSION OILS: Hyssop, Thyme, Rosemary, and Camphor

HYPO-TENSION OILS: Celery, Clary Sage, Lavender, Lemon, and Melissa

HEADACHE OILS: Grapefruit, Lavender, Melissa, Peppermint, Basil, and Eucalyptus

HEARTBURN OILS: Peppermint, German Chamomile, and Marjoram

I

INDIGESTION: Ginger, Coriander, Cardamom, Peppermint, and Lemon

INFECTION: Cinnamon, Juniper, Lavender, Lemon, Lemongrass, Black Pepper, Myrrh, Pine, and Rosemary

INFLUENZA: Ginger, Lemon, Peppermint, Black Pepper, Cinnamon, Cloves, Cypress, and Bay

INSECT REPELLANT: Citronella, Eucalyptus, Lavender, Cedarwood, Peppermint, and Sandalwood

INSOMNIA: Lavender, Clary Sage, Neroli, Petitgrain, Roman Chamomile, and Sandalwood

IRRITABILITY: Roman Chamomile, Benzoin, Geranium, Lavender, Neroli, and Sandalwood, Clary Sage

J

JET LAG: Peppermint, Rosemary, Geranium, Basil, and Grapefruit

L

LAXATIVE: Black Pepper, Ginger, Lemon, Nutmeg, Aniseed, Parsley, Rose, and Violet

LARYNGITIS: Bergamot, Cypress, Lavender, Benzoin, and Lemon

M

MEASLES: Eucalyptus, Geranium, Lavender, German Chamomile, and Bergamot

MEMORY ENHANCEMENT: Basil and Rosemary

MENOPAUSE: Clary Sage, Cypress, Geranium, Jasmine, Roman Chamomile, and Sandalwood, Lavender

MENSTRUAL PROBLEMS: Roman Chamomile, Marjoram, Clary Sage, Geranium, and Lavender

MIGRAINE: Roman Chamomile, Rosemary, Peppermint, and Lavender

MOUTH INFECTION: Tea Tree, Myrrh, and Geranium

MUMPS: Tea Tree, Lavender and German Chamomile

MUSCLE PAINS: Roman Chamomile, Clary Sage, Marjoram, Basil, Bay, Black Pepper, Peppermint, and Rosemary

N

NAUSEA: Ginger, Melissa, Clove, and Peppermint

NOSEBLEED: Cypress, Lavender, and Lemon

NEURALGIA: Black Pepper, Chamomile, Clary Sage, Bay, Benzoin, Geranium, and Peppermint

O

OVERINDULGENCE: Grapefruit, Lemon, Juniper, and Peppermint

OVER-WORK: Clary Sage, Lavender, and Neroli

P

PMS: Roman Chamomile, Clary Sage, Geranium, Neroli, and Rosemary

R

RESPIRATORY PROBLEMS: Cedarwood, Eucalyptus, Peppermint, Basil, Benzoin, Rosemary, and Sandalwood

RELAXING: Clary Sage, Geranium, Lavender, Neroli, Sandalwood, Benzoin, Carnation, and Ylang-Ylang

RHEUMATISM: Cedarwood, Chamomile, Cloves, Coriander, Eucalyptus, Lavender, Lemon, Pine, Rosemary, Black Pepper, Frankincense, and Ginger

S

SCAR TISSUE: Jasmine, Neroli, Petitgrain, Helichrysum, and Sandalwood

SEASICKNESS: Ginger

SEDATIVE: Clary Sage, Cypress, Frankincense, Jasmine, Lavender, Mandarin, Benzoin, Bergamot, Cedarwood, Melissa, Rose, Sandalwood, Ylang-Ylang, Neroli, and Petitgrain

SHOCK: Lavender and Basil

SINUSITIS: Lavender, Peppermint, Pine, Rosemary, Basil, Eucalyptus, and Tea Tree

SUNBURN: Roman Chamomile, Lavender, and Eucalyptus

T

THROAT: Eucalyptus, Lemon, Sandalwood, and Tea Tree

TONSILITIS: Tea Tree and Lavender

TOOTHACHE: Roman Chamomile, Peppermint, and Clove

TONIC: Clary Sage, Frankincense, Geranium, Ginger, Hyssop, Neroli, Orange, Pine, Rose, Rosewood, Basil, Black Pepper, Carrot Seed, Lemon, Lemongrass, Myrrh, and Nutmeg

V

VERICOSE VEINS: Lemon, Cypress, and Geranium

W

WINDBURN: Lavender and Roman Chamomile

WOUNDS: Roman Chamomile, Bergamot, Benzoin, Tea Tree, Lavender, Frankincense, and Eucalyptus

CHOOSING ESSENTIAL OILS

When selecting essential oils, you should first establish the effect the oils would have on your body, on your environment, and any safety related issues. You should also know your budget because some oils are more difficult to extract than others and, therefore, cost much more. If you find the aroma of any oil unpleasant, then you should not use the oil because your dislike for it may reduce its benefits to you. You should also know that some essential oils are not recommended for people suffering from certain conditions or falling in certain ages.

DANGEROUS ESSENTIAL OILS

The following is a list of traditional contraindications of various essential oils for specific conditions:

a. High Blood Pressure: Eucalyptus, Cypress, Rose, Ginger, Thyme, Sage and Rosemary

b. Breastfeeding: Sage, Jasmine, Parsley, and Mint

c. Pregnancy: Cinnamon, Clary Sage, Basil, Cypress, Juniper, Jasmine, Fennel, Myrrh, Marjoram, Origanum, Rose, Peppermint, Pennyroyal, Thyme, Sage, Savory, and Rosemary

d. Epilepsy: Hyssop, Rosemary, Fennel, Wormwood, and Sage

e. Low Blood Pressure: Garlic, Clary Sage, Lemon, Lavender, Marjoram, and Ylang-Ylang

f. Those who drink Alcohol: Clary Sage

g. When driving or using machinery: Vertivert and Clary Sage

HAZARDOUS ESSENTIAL OILS

The following oils MUST NEVER be used therapeutically in any way: Almond (bitter), Camphor (yellow), Camphor (brown), Boldo Leaf, Wormwood, Wormseed, Wintergreen, Plicata, Thuja, Thuja (Cedarleaf), Tansy, Southernwood, Savin, Rue, Mustard, Mugwort, Jaborandi Leaf, Horseradish, Sassafras (Brazil), and Sassafras.

The following oils MUST NEVER be used on the skin, but can be used in Fragrancers after high Dilution: Savory (winter), Pine (dwarf), Savory (summer), Origanum (Thymus capitatus), Origanum, Fennel (bitter), Elecampane, Costus, Cinnamon Bark, Clove Stem, Clove Leaf, Clove Buds, and Cassia.

Chapter 8: Essential Oils Recipes and Blends for Treating Specific Medical Conditions

1. Relieving Abdominal Pain

For relieving abdominal pain, blend 5ml carrier oil with 1 drop of Chamomile, 1 drop of Clove Oil, and 1 drop of Peppermint oil, and massage the stomach area gently with the blend.

2. Relieving Abscess Induced Pain

Prepare a compress using 2 drops of Tea Tree, 2 drops of Chamomile, and 2 drops of Lavender, and apply the compress to the swollen area twice a day.

3. Treating Acne

Acne can be treated by applying a few drops of diluted Tea Tree or diluted Lavender to the individual marks every night, until the marks disappear. A more potent acne preparation can be made by blending Benzoin, Lavender, Cedarwood, German Chamomile, Geranium,

Tea Tree Oil, and a suitable carrier (such as Jojoba oil) with dilutions for oil (the oils used in the blend not exceeding 2%).

4. Overcoming Addictions

If you want to overcome certain bad habits, then you should massage your body, inhale, or take baths using essential oils, like Lavender, Jasmine, Ylang-Ylang, Bergamot, Roman Chamomile, or Clary Sage.

5. Treating Anal Fissures

Add 1 drop of Lemon oil and 1 drop of Lavender oil to warm water and then bathe the anal fissures in the water.

6. Preventing and Treating Athlete's Foot

To prevent the condition, add and rub a few drops of Geranium oil or Tea Tree oil inside the shoe before and after wearing. The oils should be diluted.

To treat infected feet, blend 2 drops of Tea Tree oil, 2 drops of Geranium oil, and 2 drops of Wheat Germ oil with 10 ml carrier oil and rub the oil blend around the nails and between the toes every day.

7. Preventing Bad Breath

Prepare a mouthwash for bad breath by mixing 4 drops of Lavender oil with 5 ml Brandy and 125 ml warm water and swirl the mixture in the mouth after proper flossing and brushing. Then, spit it out and rinse your mouth properly.

8. Treating Bedsores

Make massage oil for bedsores by blending 20 ml carrier oil (like Evening Primrose Oil), 2 drops Frankincense oil, 2 drops Tea Tree oil, 2 drops Lavender oil, 4 drops of Wheat Germ oil, and 3 drops Chamomile (or Geranium oil). After mixing the ingredients, massage the affected areas gently.

9. Stopping Bleeding

To stop blood loss during emergency or accident, apply a compress to the small open wound (s). The compress used should be made with 1 drop Tea Tree oil, 1 drop Chamomile oil, 1 drop Lemon oil, and 1 drop Geranium oil.

10. Treating Bleeding Gums

Bleeding gums are treated using mouthwash. Make the mouthwash by blending the following oils: 3 drops Thyme oil, 3 drops Peppermint oil, 3 drops Chamomile oil, and 2 drops Eucalyptus oil and diluting them in 1 tablespoonful of Brandy. Add the resulting blend to warm water and swirl it in the mouth for 5-10 minutes. Do not swallow the mouthwash. Visit a dentist if the problem persists.

11. Treating Blepharitis

Blepharitis is the inflammation of the outer edge of the eyelid. It can cause itching, redness, burning, or a sensation of having something in the eye. To treat blepharitis, prepare a compress by mixing 1 drop Chamomile oil with 5ml Witch Hazel and then adding the mixture into 30ml Rosewater. Leave the blend for at least 7 hours and apply it on closed eyelids.

12. Treating Blisters

Apply 1-2 drops of Lavender oil and 1 drop of Chamomile oil to the blister and pat it gently.

13. Treating Boils

Bathe the affected area 2 times a day using a blend of 2 drops Lavender oil, 1 drop Juniper, 2 drops Tea Tree oil, and 200ml hot water. If you experience severe inflammation, it is advisable to add 1 drop of Chamomile oil as one of the ingredients.

14. Relieving Breathing Difficulties

Prepare massage oil using 5 drops Nutmeg oil, 10 drops Eucalyptus oil, 2 drops Cinnamon oil, 10 drops Ginger oil, 3 drops Rosemary oil, and 30 ml Carrier oil. Rub the massage oil gently around the back and chest. For acute breathing problems, use steam inhalation with Hyssop oil or Eucalyptus oil. But for chronic conditions, prepare massage oil of 15 drops Eucalyptus oil, 10 drops Rosemary oil, 5 drops Hyssop oil, and 30 ml carrier oil, and massage the back, neck, and chest with the resulting massage oil.

15. Treating Bronchitis

To ease your breathing, try inhaling any of the following essential oils: Basil, Benzoin, Pine, Clove, Tea Tree, or Frankincense. You can also vaporize a mixture of 15 drops Eucalyptus oil and 5 drops of Oregano oil in 600 ml warm water and inhale.

16. Treating Bruises

If you want to enhance the healing of bruises, massage the affected area with Lavender oil. You can also use massage oil made of 5 drops Calendula oil, 2 drops Fennel oil, 1 drop Cypress oil, and 10ml Grape seed oil.

17. Treating Minor Burns

Apply 1-2 drops of Lavender to the burns and cover with a damp compress. Seek professional attention quickly.

18. Treating Carbuncles

Bathe affected area with a blend of 2 drops Tea Tree oil and 2 drops Lavender oil diluted in 125ml hot water.

19. Treating Catarrh

Add 1 drop of Thyme oil and 1 drop of Eucalyptus oil to a bowl of hot water. Cover your head with a towel and inhale the aroma for 10 minutes. A bath of Eucalyptus oil is also effective. You can also prepare massage oil of 15 ml Evening Primrose oil, 3 drops Eucalyptus oil, 3 drops Rosemary oil, and 3 drops Tea Tree oil and rub the oil on the back and chest areas.

20. Treating Chapped Lips

To ease the pain on the chapped lips and boost healing, prepare a blend oil of 2 drops Rose oil, 1 drop Neroli oil, 2 drops Geranium oil, 1 drop Chamomile oil, and 20 ml Aloe Vera oil and apply the blend on the chapped lips.

21. Combating Chilblains

Apply 1-3 drops of Geranium, Tea Tree or Lemon Juice to the affected part (usually fingers or toes). A more potent option is a blend oil of 2 drops Tea Tree oil, 2 drops Black Pepper oil, 2 drops Lavender oil, 2 drops Geranium oil, and 10 ml Calendula infused oil.

22. Boosting Blood Circulation

Prepare massage oil using 2 drops Cypress oil, 2 drops Neroli oil, 2 drops Lemon oil, and 2 drops Geranium oil into 15ml carrier oil. Massage the affected areas using the oil blend.

23. Treating Constipation

Prepare massage oil using 15 drops Rosemary oil, 10 drops Lemon oil, and 5 drops Peppermint oil into 30 ml Jojoba oil and apply the blend to the lower abdomen 3 times a day.

24. Treating Conjunctivitis

To treat sore itchy eyes, cover them with a compress soaked in chamomile or fennel oil. And, to treat conjunctivitis, prepare a compress using 1 drop chamomile oil, 5ml Witch hazel, and 30ml Rosewater and apply the compress to closed eyelids.

25. Safeguarding Homes and Offices against Flu and Colds

Prepare a spray by adding 1 drop Cinnamon oil, 1 drop Cloves oil, 1 drop Eucalyptus oil, 1 drop Niaouli oil, and 1 drop Pine oil into 500ml water. Add the blend into a spray bottle, shake well, and spray the home or office. To relieve the stuffiness of colds, prepare blends of Cajuput, Clove, Eucalyptus, Niaouli, and Pine into an inhaler, bath, or handkerchief.

26.Relieving Cold Sores

Use Geranium, Chamomile, or Calendula oil to relieve the swelling and pain.

27.Relieving Coughs

Drink an expectorant made of properly diluted Thyme, Lavender, Mint, Melissa, or Rosewater. You can also use steam inhalation of Eucalyptus oil or sip 1 teaspoonful of a mixture of 2 drops eucalyptus oil, 2 drops lemon oil, and 3 tablespoonfuls of honey. Besides, coughs can be relieved by massaging the back and chest using massage oil made from 3 drops of eucalyptus oil, 1 drop pine oil, 2 drops thyme oil, and 1 teaspoonful jojoba oil.

28.Treating Cuts

Prepare a blend for washing and cleaning the cut by using 500ml water, 2 drops Tea Tree oil, 1 drop

Eucalyptus oil, and 4 drops Lavender. Using the blend, wash the cut gently. If you want to sterilize the wound, you can use Lemon oil as an emergency wound sterilizer (though it stings).

29. Treating Diarrhea

Prepare and drink Ginger tea to treat abdominal cramps and pains. And, to stop the diarrhea, prepare massage oil using 2 drops peppermint, 2 drops lavender, 2 drops chamomile, 2 drops geranium, and 2 drops eucalyptus in 10 ml carrier oil. Apply the oil to the abdomen and rub gently.

30. Relieving Diverticulitis

Prepare massage oil by blending 1 drop peppermint, 1 drop chamomile, 2 drops rosemary, and 1 drop clove oil into 5 ml carrier oil. Rub the massage oil on the stomach in clockwise motion to ease the discomfort.

31. Treating Dysmenorrhea (Painful Menstruation)

Prepare herbal tea using aniseed, parsley, or fennel to relieve the pain. You can also create an effective massage oil using 1 drop peppermint oil, 2 drops lavender oil, 2 drops geranium, 2 drops clary sage, 2 drops bay oil, and 15 ml jojoba base oil. Using the blend, massage the painful area gently.

32. Treating Ear Infection and Earache

To relieve earache, blend 1 drop clove oil with 5 ml grape seed oil and massage the area around the ear and neck with the blend. But, if the ear infection is caused by throat infection, you should add 2 drops of Tea Tree oil to a glass of boiled water and gargle after every 2 hours.

33. Relieving Fainting

Help the patient to regain consciousness by holding open a bottle of Rosemary, Lavender, or Peppermint oil over the patient's nose to let the patient inhale the oil's vapor.

34. Relieving Fever

Make herbal tea with eucalyptus, chamomile, thyme, and rosemary and drink warm with honey. You can also relieve the fever by massaging the top of hands, back of neck, temples, and soles of feet, using a blend of oil combining 1 drop of rosemary, 1 drop of tea tree, 1 drop of black pepper, 2 drops of peppermint, 2 drops of lavender, and 2 drops of eucalyptus into 15 ml Evening Primrose oil.

35. Treating Flu

Firstly, you can drink herbal teas (tisanes) made of thyme, hyssop, eucalyptus, and chamomile. Secondly, you can add 4 drops of tea tree oil, 3 drops of lavender, and 1 drop of lemon oil into warm water and have a warm bath to lift your body. After the bath, you can apply massage oil made of 10ml evening primrose oil, 3 drops of tea tree oil and 2 drops of eucalyptus oil. Finally, you can vaporize the room using lavender, clove and pine oil to ease flu symptoms.

36. Treating Frostbite

Apply a few drops of lavender to the patches of affected skin. And at the end of your day, add a few drops of cypress and pine oil to your feet or as massage oil.

37. Relieving Gingivitis

Prepare a mouthwash for gingivitis by adding 3 drops of Thyme oil, 2 drops of Eucalyptus oil, 3 drops of Chamomile oil, and 3 drops of Peppermint oil into 1 tablespoonful Brandy. Add the mixture into a glass of warm water and swish well around the mouth. Do not swallow the mouthwash.

38.Treating Grazes

Prepare a bathing solution using 10 drops of eucalyptus, lavender, tea tree, or lemon oil into a bowl of warm water.

39.Treating Halitosis

To achieve better smelling breath, you can chew herbs such as mint, cinnamon, parsley or thyme. Moreover, you can fight halitosis by adding 1 drop of Myrrh oil to 1 cup of boiled water and using as a mouthwash.

40.Treating Hay Fever

Drink tisanes made from eucalyptus leaves, rosehips, or pine needles. Secondly, you can add a few drops of tea tree, Niaouli, or eucalyptus oil on your handkerchief and use when attacked. Moreover, you can boil eucalyptus leaves in water and make a room/bedroom spray with the resulting liquid.

41.Treating Headache

For relieving headache, you should prepare massage oil by mixing 3 drops lavender oil, 1 drop peppermint oil, 1 drop bergamot oil, and 3 drops jojoba oil, and using the blend to massage the base of your skull or the area around the temples. But, if you have a nervous or tension headache, then you should prepare and use a blend of 3 drops of lavender oil, 1 drop of clary sage, 1 drop of chamomile, and 2 drops of jojoba oil.

42.Treating Heart Palpitations

Drink tisanes of cooling plants, such as lime, basil, chamomile, orange leaves, or Melissa. You can also inhale lavender oil.

43.Relieving Heartburn

Prepare massage oil using 2 drops eucalyptus oil, 1 drop peppermint oil, 2 drops fennel oil, and 5ml (1 teaspoonful) grape seed oil and rub the blend oil on the upper abdominal area.

44. Relieving Hiccups

Add 1 drop of Chamomile oil into a brown paper bag and hold over your mouth and nose, breathe in the aroma deeply and slowly.

45. Treating High Blood Pressure

A relaxing massage can help to lower blood pressure. Essential oils that are effective for high blood pressure are Clary Sage, Melissa, Ylang-Ylang, Marjoram, and Lavender. Remember to avoid using the following essential oils if you have high blood pressure, Hyssop (contains pinocamphone), Sage (contains thujone), Thyme (hypertensive), and Rosemary (very stimulating).

46. Treating Influenza

Make and drink tisanes using eucalyptus, chamomile, thyme, and hyssop to restore fluids lost due to influenza fever. Secondly, you should safeguard your office or house using a spray made of a blend of 1 drop pine oil, 1 drop Niaouli oil, 1 drop eucalyptus oil, 1 drop cloves oil, and 1 drop cinnamon oil into 500 ml water. Thirdly, you can relieve the stuffiness of influenza colds by inhaling, massaging, or bathing in a blend of cajuput, pine, eucalyptus, Niaouli, and cloves oil.

47.Relieving Insect Bites (ticks, fleas and spiders)

Remove the sting by applying a few drops of Lavender or Chamomile to the bite area.

48.Repelling Insects

Use the following essential oils either individually or as a blend: citronella oil (very good for mosquitoes), peppermint, lavender, thyme, and lemongrass oil.

49.Relieving Insomnia

Perform a relaxing massage using clary sage, sandalwood, lavender, Petitgrain or ylang-ylang mixed with suitable carrier oil.

50.Relieving Jetlag

Massage your feet during the flight with a few drops of diluted geranium, basil, or grapefruit. On arrival, you can boost your alertness by rubbing 10 drops of lavender on your torso and then showering properly. Moreover, you can revive your mind and body by adding 2 drops of peppermint, 1 drop of rosemary, 1 drop of bergamot, 2 drops of neroli, and 1 drop of geranium into warm water and taking a warm refreshing bath.

51. Treating Laryngitis

Add 2 drops of cajuput, geranium, black pepper, or rosemary into a glass of cooled boiled water and gargle 5-6 times a day. Steam inhalation of 2 drops lavender, 1 drop thyme, 1 drop eucalyptus, and 1 drop chamomile in heated water can also relieve laryngitis.

52. Relieving Leg Cramps

Prepare massage oil of 3 drops geranium into 5 ml evening primrose oil and rub the massage oil vigorously on the legs until the cramp is relieved.

53. Treating Lumbago

Add 3 drops of oregano, rosemary, or thyme oil to your bath and soak yourself for at least 20 minutes. You can also prepare and use massage oil containing 3 drops rosemary oil, 1 drop eucalyptus oil, 2 drops peppermint oil, 2 drops chamomile oil, and 1 drop cardamom oil into 10 ml evening primrose oil. Using the massage oil, massage the lower back down to the top end of your buttocks. Avoid the anus because it has sensitive membranes that may be irritated.

54. Treating Mouth Ulcers

Apply a cotton bud that has been dipped in Tea Tree oil to the ulcer for immediate relief. You can also prepare and use a mouthwash of 5ml salt and 2 drops Tea Tree oil into 500 ml warm boiled water.

55. Relieving Nausea

Add a few drops of bergamot or lavender oil to a handkerchief and sniff it to relieve motion sickness.

56. Treating Neuralgia

Prepare massage oil by blending 1 drop clove oil, 3 drops black pepper oil, 3 drops chamomile oil, and 3 drops lavender oil into 10 ml grape seed oil. Massage the blend into the spot.

57.Preventing Shock

Prepare message oil by mixing 3 drops lemon oil, 2 drops geranium oil, 2 drops lavender oil, 1 drop German chamomile oil, and 1 drop Petitgrain oil into 20 ml carrier oil. Massage the entire body with the oil blend just before retiring to bed.

58.Relieving Pneumonia

Drink tisanes made from thyme, oregano or eucalyptus herbal material. Another option is steam inhalation of cypress or pine oil.

59.Stopping Nosebleed

Pinch the nostrils and then inhale a blend of 3 drops lemon oil and 1 drop lavender oil. An icepack made of lemon oil and lavender oil can also be effective. If the nosebleed is due to an injured or broken nose, you should see your doctor immediately.

60.Treating Sinusitis

Prepare and use steam inhalation of a blend of 2 drops rosemary oil, 2 drops peppermint oil, 1 drop thyme oil, and 1 drop eucalyptus oil. After steam inhalation, you should prepare massage oil, using 1 drop tea tree oil, 3 drops geranium oil, 3 drops rosemary oil, 2 drops peppermint oil, and 2 drops eucalyptus oil. Then, massage the oil on the forehead, cheekbones, around the nose and neck, and behind the ears.

61.Relieving Sore Throat

To relieve the discomfort caused by sore throat, prepare massage oil using 4 drops chamomile oil, 1 drop thyme oil, 1 drop lemon oil, and 1 drop tea tree oil into 5 ml carrier oil. Apply the massage oil to the neck and areas towards the back of the ears and rub thoroughly. Besides, steam inhalation of a blend of 2 drops lavender, 2 drops eucalyptus, and 1 drop thyme oil into hot water can be helpful.

62.Relieving Sties

Add 1 drop chamomile to 10ml rosewater and boil well before cooling and filtering using a coffee filter. Use the strained liquid to create a compress and then use the compress on the affected eye.

63.Treating Swollen Ankles

Prepare massage oil for swollen eyes by blending 15 drops fennel oil and 15 drops of cypress oil into 30 ml evening primrose oil. Use the oil blend to massage the feet up to the knees.

64.Relieving Toothache

Add a few drops of clove oil on a cotton bud and apply into the crevices and gum of the aching tooth. You can also prepare and use massage oil containing 1 drop clove oil, 3 drops chamomile oil, and 1 drop lemon oil into 5 ml carrier oil. Apply the oil blend on the cheek and jawbone, massaging gently.

65.Relieving Varicose Veins

Prepare massage oil by adding 4 drops cypress oil, 4 drops lavender oil, and 2 drops wheat germ oil into 20 ml almond oil. Apply the massage oil to the legs and feet and massage gently every day to relieve the pain.

66.Treating Wounds

Add 5 drops lavender oil and 2 drops tea tree oil into 500 ml warm water and bathe the wound area. You can also cover up the wound, using a piece of gauze onto which 3 drops of lavender oil has been added.

67.Essential Oils for Skin and Beauty

A number of essential oils can be used to create effective skin care and beauty products. Here are specific oils you can consider for different conditions:

a. Reducing age spots: Frankincense

b. Thickening hair: Sage and Rosemary

c. Calming irritated skin: Roman Chamomile and Lavender

d. Improving acne: Geranium and Melaleuca (Tea Tree)

e. Natural SPF skin protection: Myrrh and Helichrysum

67.Essential Oils for Hair Growth

The use of essential oils on your hair can help you prevent or stop hair loss. Oils, such as Lavender, Sage, and Rosemary, can help you to stimulate hair thickening naturally by stimulating hair follicles. Lavender and Clary Sage support hair growth by promoting the balance of estrogen levels while Rosemary essential oil boosts hair growth by inhibiting DHT (di-hydroxy-testosterone), which prevents hair loss.

To thicken your hair naturally, add 10 drops of Rosemary and 5 drops of Lavender to different sections of your scalp and massage the oils into your scalp for 2 minutes. Cover your head with a hot towel for 20 minutes and then wash the hair with a natural homemade shampoo.

68. Essential Oil Bug Spray

Mosquitoes and bugs can ruin vacations, special occasions, and BBQs and should therefore be kept away using effective sprays. Homemade natural bug sprays containing essential oils are safe and do not contain toxic chemicals, such as DEET. Here are the best essential oils to use in insect-repelling bug sprays:

(i) Eucalyptus

(ii)   Clove

(iii)   Peppermint

(iv)   Citronella

(v)   Lemongrass

(vi)   Geranium

(vii)   Rosemary

You can spray or rub any of these essential oils on your body to repel the bugs. However, because of different species of bugs, you should blend two or more essential oils to create more potent repellants.

69. Essential Oils for Weight Loss

Doing the right exercises and improving your diet can help you to lose weight. But if you require an extra boost in achieving your weight loss goals quickly, then certain essential oils are ideal for you. The following essential oils are effective in burning fat:

(i)   Peppermint suppresses cravings and boosts digestion.

(ii) Cinnamon balances blood sugar levels and assists in weight loss; it also helps in improving diabetes.

(iii) Ginger Oil contains Gingerol, which increases thermogenesis and boosts metabolism.

(iv) Grapefruit Oil contains d-Limonene, which improves the secretion of metabolic enzymes.

16. Essential oils for Natural First Aid Kit

Assembling a homemade First Aid Kit is an ideal preparation for potential wounds, sunburns, stings, muscle pain, or injury. Here are some essential oils that you should keep in you medicine cabinet as part of your First Aid Kit:

a. Lavender: Used for healing burns, stings, rashes, cuts, reducing anxiety and helping you to sleep after trauma.
b. Frankincense: Used to heal bruising, reduce scars, anti-inflammatory, boost immunity, and promote emotional well-being.
c. Malaleuca (Tea Tree): Used as anti-bacterial, antifungal, and antiseptic. It cleans air of

allergens and pathogens and prevents/reduces infection.

d. Peppermint: Relieves muscle and joint pain, reduces fevers, clears sinuses, relieves headaches, improves digestive problems, and relieves bronchitis and asthma.

e. Cypress: Treating sore throat and varicose veins.

f. Eucalyptus: Treating colds, flu, shingles, inflammation, and congestion.

g. German Chamomile: Relieving bruises, sprains, and inflammation.

h. Sweet Marjoram: For soothing menstrual cramps, helping with insomnia, and relieving sore muscles.

i. Spearmint: Helping with sinusitis, fever, indigestion, and poison ivy.

j. Rosemary: Improves aches, fatigue, hangover, constipation, and poor circulation.

k. Orange: Helps with depression, digestion, and lymphatic congestion.

17. Using Essential Oils for Home and Hearth

a. Deterring Pests: Use lavender for getting rid of moths and mosquitoes.

b. Keeping Humidifiers Clean: Add 9 drops of Tea Tree oil (has antimicrobial properties) into the humidifier.

c. Perfumed Fire Logs: Add a few drops of cedarwood, sandalwood, pine, or cypress oil to a log 30 minutes before burning the log in fire.

d. Soothing Kids with Stuffed Animals: Placed a stuffed animal into a plastic bag containing a few drops of essential oil and close the plastic bag overnight. The next day, the stuffed animal will have the scent of the oil and will disperse it in air for up to 2 weeks.

Chapter 9: SAFETY CONSIDERATIONS WHEN USING ESSENTIAL OILS

Safety refers to the state of being free from the risk or occurrence of danger, harm, or injury. All individuals intending to use essential oils should be aware of the safety issues involved, so they can avoid potential adverse effects of the oils. In fact, while essential oils are potentially dangerous materials, the risks involved in using them are significantly very small if they are handled in appropriate manner. Indeed, while informed and careful use of essential oils may not prevent the occasional irritation and minor discomfort that may occur, it is highly unlikely that essential oils will cause serious physical problems or injury, if used cautiously.

FACTORS INFLUENCING ESSENTIAL OIL SAFETY

a. Quality of the essential oil being used: Using pure, genuine, and authentic essential oils reduces the likelihood of adverse effects, but adulterated oils may cause significant health problems.

b. Chemical composition of the essential oil: Oils rich in phenols and aldehydes may cause skin reactions. To reduce risks involved, dilute the oils as recommended.

c. Method of application: Essential oils may be applied topically on the skin, inhaled, taken internally, or diffused. Every application method comes with its safety issues.

d. Dilution/dosage to be applied: Most essential oils are usually diluted between 1% and 5%, reducing safety issues significantly. Excessive use of essential oils or using high concentration may result in irritation and sensitization.

e. Integrity of the skin: Inflamed, damaged, or diseased skin will be more permeable and more sensitive to essential oils. Therefore, do not apply undiluted essential oils on inflamed, damaged, or diseased skin.

f. Age of the user: Infants, toddlers, and young children are more sensitive than adults to the potency of essential oils. Therefore, safe dilutions for young children, toddlers, and infants are 0.5%-2.5%. Similarly, elderly users can experience more skin sensitivities than other adults, and the concentration of the oils they use should be reduced as necessary.

POSSIBLE DERMAL REACTIONS TO ESSENTIAL OILS

The possible dermal (skin) reactions that may occur after using essential oils include sensitization, irritation, and photosensitization (phototoxicity).

a. **Dermal Irritation:** Dermal irritants usually cause redness, blotchiness, and severe pain on the skin, and the severity of the reactions depend on the concentration (dilution) of the essential oil applied. To avoid irritation, it is important not to use known irritants on allergic or sensitive skin; dilute the irritants properly; perform skin patch test; and avoid applying the dermal irritants on damaged or open skin. Common skin irritants include: Bay (Pimento racemosa), Cinnamon bark/leaf (Cinnamomum zeylanicum), Clove Bud (Syzygium aromaticum), Citronella

(Cymbopogon nardus), Cumin (Cuminum cyminum), Lemongrass (Cymbopogon citratus), Lemon verbena (Lippia citriodora), Oregano (Origanum vulgare), Tagetes (Tagetes minuta), and Thyme ct. thymol (Thymus vulgaris).

b. **Dermal Sensitization:** Skin sensitization is an allergic reaction occurring normally after first exposure to an essential oil, which results in minor or no noticeable effect. But, it leads to severe inflammation during subsequent exposure to the same essential oil. Ideally, the first exposure leads to the formation of T-lymphocytes against the oil, resulting in blotchiness, redness, and pain during subsequent exposure. To avoid sensitization, essential oils should be diluted thoroughly and the same essential oil must never be applied every day for an extended period of time. Dermal sensitizers should also be avoided. Common dermal sensitizers include Cinnamon bark, Peru Balsam, Cassia oil, Verbana absolute, Inula, Backhousia, Turpentine oil, and Tea absolute.

c. **Photosensitization:** Photosensitive essential oils cause skin pigmentation changes (like tanning) and burning when exposed to sunlight (ultraviolet rays). To avoid photosensitization, such essential oils must not be used prior to going into the sun or san tanning booth. Commonly used photosensitive essential oils include Angelica root (Angelica archangelica), Cumin (Cuminum cyminum), Bergamot (Citrus bergamia), Expressed Lime (Citrus medica), Expressed Lemon (Citrus limon), expressed Bitter Orange (Citrus aurantium), and Rue (Ruta Graveolens). Instead of the photosensitive (phototoxic) essential oils, non-phototoxic essential oils, such as Distilled lemon, Distilled Lime, Sweet Orange, Yuzu oil, and Furanocoumarin-Free Bergamot, should be used.

d. Mucous Membrane Irritation and Sensitization

Essential oils that produce drying or heating effects on the mucous membranes of the eyes, mouth, reproductive organs, and nose are called Mucous Membrane Irritants. Such essential oils should never be used in full body baths except when first placed in dispersants, such as vegetable oil or milk. Irritants, such as Bay, Lemongrass, Cinnamon bark, Thyme ct. thymol, and clove oil, should be completely avoided in baths. Common essential oils that irritate mucous membranes are Bay, Caraway, Cinnamon bark (leaf), Lemongrass, Clove leaf (bud), Peppermint, and Thyme ct. thymol.

SAFETY CONSIDERATIONS DURING PREGNANCY/BREASTFEEDING

Usage of essential oils during pregnancy constitutes a huge risk to the fetus, especially during the first 3-month period. While there is no evidence that inhalation or topical application of essential oils by pregnant women have ever caused miscarriages, birth defects, or abnormal fetuses, experts agree that toxicity during pregnancy will occur if the woman takes large doses of essential oils. Nevertheless, judicious use of essential oils in the form of massages by skilled therapists is encouraged for pregnant women, as it can ease discomforts and help pregnant women to develop a nurturing attitude towards their unborn babies. Here are safety guidelines for using essential oils during pregnancy:

a. Do not apply essential oils internally when you are pregnant.

b. Avoid undiluted application of essential oils when you are pregnant.

c. Use essential oils that are generally classified as safe, such as Roman Chamomile, German chamomile, Cardamom, Geranium, Ginger, Frankincense, Petitgrain, Rose, Rosewood, Patchouli, Neroli, and Sandalwood.

d. Avoid the following oils: Rue, Wormwood, Camphor, Sage, Hyssop, Parsley seed, Aniseed, Basil ct. estragole, Pennyroyal, Oak Moss, Thuja, Wintergreen, and Lavandula.

GENERAL SAFETY CONSIDERATIONS FOR ESSENTIAL OILS

a. Do not buy or use essential oils that you know nothing about. Research and get to know more about any essential oil before buying it.

b. Avoid prolonged use of the same essential oils.

c. Keep all essential oils away/out of the reach of pets and children.

d. Never use photosensitive essential oils prior to sun exposure. If you apply such oils on your skin, stay away from the sun for at least 24 hours.

e. Dilute all essential oils before applying to your skin, unless indicated otherwise.

f. If you have a treatment room where you use essential oils, make sure that it has good ventilation.

g. If you suspect sensitivity or allergy to certain essential oils, perform skin patch test before using the oil.

h. Essential oils are typically highly flammable substances which must be kept away from direct flames, fire, candles, gas cookers, matches, and cigarettes.

i. Keep and use essential oils away from the eyes.

j. Essential oils must be chosen carefully and used with caution on the immuno-compromised, persons with chronic conditions, children, elderly, pregnant women, and nursing mothers.

k. Essential oils must never be ingested (used internally) unless under the guidance and supervision of trained aromatherapy expert.

l. If essential oil droplets get into the eye (s) accidentally, then a cotton cloth should be imbued with fatty oil (like sesame or olive) and swiped carefully over the closed lid. After that, the eyes should be flushed with cold water.

m. In case of dermal irritation, a small amount of vegetable oil should be applied to the affected area and the use of the dermal irritant should be discontinued immediately.

n. If a child drinks several spoonfuls of essential oils, contact the nearest poison control unit immediately. Meanwhile, the child should be given whole or 2% milk, but not encouraged to vomit.

CHAPTER 10: HOW TO BUY ESSENTIAL OILS

Quality essential oils have the capacity to restore health and wellness and to solve a number of common problems. Unfortunately, the essential oils market is replete with poor quality oils that have been diluted with cheap low-grade oils or cheaper substitutes and synthetic fragrances. Still, if you want to buy best quality essential oils, then you should make your purchases from a reputable supplier. Below are top tips to remember when buying essential oils:

a. Do not confuse perfume oils with essential oils. Perfume oils do not give the same therapeutic benefits as essential oils.

b. Do not buy essential oils stored in rubber glass dropper tops as essential oils are highly concentrated and will convert the rubber to gum and ruin the oil.

c. Do not buy essential oils before reading as much information as possible about them and consulting naturopathic experts. Reading and consulting experts will help you to master the safety issues involved in using essential oils, so you can maximize their benefits.

d. Do not buy essential oils from just any aromatherapy store or company. The quality of essential oils varies significantly from one manufacturer to another. Some companies also claim their oils are pure or can be used undiluted, when the oils are not. Buy from a trusted supplier.

e. Do not search for essential oils by using their common names such as bay, cedarwood, anise, lavender, and eucalyptus. There are many different varieties of each of the essential oil plants and the common names would lead you to the wrong oils. Instead, search for the essential oils using their Latin names (botanical names). For instance, Bay essential oil is a common name for either Pimenta racemosa or Laurus nobilis.

f. Check for the country of origin of essential oils you intend to buy before buying them. Most honest suppliers of the oils usually provide the botanical name and country of origin. Similarly, you should pay attention to whether the oil is organic, ethically farmed, or wild-crafted.

g. If you are buying essential oils for the first time or just beginning to use them, do not purchase the oils from vendors on craft shows, street fairs, and other limited-time events. You should always have enough time to judge the quality of the oil you are buying.

h. Purchasing essential oils from reputable and experienced mail-order suppliers/companies can help you to obtain higher quality oil inexpensively than when you buy from a generic local health and food store.

i. Make sure to pay special attention to the safety information on the essential oil labels. And, if you have any medical condition or are pregnant, then you must be extra careful with the quality, purity, types, and safety of oils you use.

j. Store essential oils in dark glass (cobalt blue or amber glass) and in a cool and dark place.

You can find reputable essential oil suppliers on the high street or online. To do so:

(i)   You must be very cautious of less-known suppliers who use phrases such as "therapeutic grade" or "aromatherapy grade" on their oil bottles in order to sell their products. The supplier or company you choose should be well-known and must have a good reputation.

(ii)   You should know that reputable suppliers or companies usually sell their essential oils in small colored bottles; while sellers of low-quality and "fake" essential oils often use clear bottles and offer larger quantities. A high quality essential oil must come in a colored bottle of around four liquid ounces or smaller.

(iii)   You should use the Internet to find information about reputable essential oil suppliers and who to avoid. A simple and quick Google search can lead you to several aromatherapy websites, blogs, forums, and communities dedicated to discussing and promoting best quality essential oils.

CONCLUSION

Essential oils are natural therapeutic agents for many common health problems. They contain chemical components that can alter the functions and structure of body cells, resulting in nourishing, grounding, relaxing, or healing effects. Nevertheless, since the chemical components are highly concentrated in the oils, it is advisable to dilute all essential oils before usage, unless indicated otherwise by a naturopathic doctor.

Besides, since essential oils are obtained from plant materials, they come with risks of allergic reactions. In fact, even an essential oil that has been used previously without adverse reactions may cause negative effects during subsequent exposure. Therefore, the use of essential oils must be based on common sense, the principals of natural therapeutics, and informed decision making. Indeed, no one should buy and use a new essential oil product without first researching and understanding the components of the product and the possible safety issues. The more you know, the more you will be successful with essential oils.

Finally, when starting out to use essential oils, it is important to start with just one or two oils, master how to use them well, and then build your collection gradually. This way, you will have the time to test and experiment with the essential oils, one after another, and to comprehend the safety issues involved more clearly.